INTERMITTENT FASTING FOR WOMEN

How To Lose Weight, Increase Energy, Boost Metabolism And Detox Your Body By Living A Long And Healthy Life.

Includes Weekly Meal Plan.

By

GRETA GREEN

The data gave in this is expressed, to be honest, and predictable, in that any risk, as far as absentmindedness or something else, by any utilization or maltreatment of any approaches, procedures, or bearings contained inside is the singular and articulate obligation of the beneficiary per user. By no means will any lawful obligation or fault be held against the distributor for any reparation, harms, or money related misfortune because of the data in this, either straightforwardly or by implication.

Particular creators claim all copyrights not held by the distributor.

The data in this is offered for educational purposes exclusively and is all-inclusive as so. The introduction of the data is without a contract or any sort of assurance confirmation.

The trademarks that are utilized are with no assent, and the distribution of the trademark is without consent or support by the trademark proprietor. All trademarks and brands inside this book are for explaining purposes just and are simply possessed by the proprietors, not partnered with this record.

TABLE OF CONTENTS

WHAT IS INTERMITTENT FASTING?

Intermittent fasting is a cycle between fasting and eating times. It is currently a standard method of weight loss and health improvement. In the New England Journal of Medicine, it was not only the "trendiest" term for weight loss quest in 2019, but it was also prominently mentioned in a summary paper.

But fasting is nothing "new." Indeed, intermittent fasting may be an ancient health secret. It is old because it was taught in the history of humankind. This is a secret because this potentially strong practice has been virtually forgotten about our wellbeing until recently.

Today, however, several people are rediscovering this dietary practice. Since 2010, the amount of online "intermediate fasting" searches has increased by approximately 10,000 percent, with the most growth in recent years. Intermittent fasting may have significant health benefits if appropriately performed, including excess weight loss, type 2 diabetes care and many other things. Moreover, it will save you money and time. The purpose of this beginner's guide is to provide everything you need to know about intermittent fasting to start.

What is fasting intermittently? Intermittent fasting – isn't it hunger? No. Fasting differs from hunger in one primary way: power. Hunger is the accidental shortage of food for a long time. This could lead to severe suffering or even death. It is neither conscious nor managed.

On the other hand, fasting requires voluntary abstinence of food for social, nutritional or other purposes. This is achieved by a person who is not underweight and therefore has enough body fat stored to live off. Intermittent fasting done right does not cause pain or death.

Food is good to eat, but you should not like it. It can take a couple of hours, a couple of days or even a week or so – with professional supervision. You can start quickly and finish at will at any time of your choosing. You can start or stop fast or for no reason.

Fasting has no traditional length, as it is merely a lack of food. Whenever you don't eat, you fast intermittently. For example, you can easily spend around 12-14 hours between dinner and breakfast the next day. Intermittent fasting should also be considered as a part of daily life.

Maybe it is the oldest and most effective food procedure imaginable. Take the term "breakfast." This refers to the meal that breaks fast every day. Instead of any kind of cruel and unusual punishment, the English language accepts that fasting, except for a short time, should be done every day.

Intermittent fasting is not an unusual and curious thing but a part of everyday life. Maybe it is the oldest and most effective dietary technique imaginable. Nevertheless, we have somehow underestimated its power and ignored its therapeutic value.

Intermittent Fasting For Losing Weight

At the very heart of intermittent fasting, the body may use its retained energy, for example, by consuming off extra body fat. This is natural, and for shorter periods of hours or days, humans have multiplied without adverse health consequences. Body fat is all food resources locked away. If the body doesn't feed, it actually "eats" its energy fat.

Life is about harmony. Life is about harmony. The good ones and the bad ones, the yin and the yang. The same goes for Diet and fasting. After all, fasting is just the flip side of food. If you don't eat, you fast. That is how it functions: As we feed, more energy is absorbed than can be used instantly. Some of this energy needs to be stored to be used later. Insulin is the primary hormone involved in food energy production.

When we eat, insulin rises to help us store extra sugar in two different ways. The glucose (sugar) units of carbohydrates can be bound to long chains to form glycogen, which then is stored in the liver or muscle. Nevertheless, carbohydrates have very little storage space, and once that has been exceeded, the liver begins to make surplus glucose fat. It is called de-novo lipogenesis (meaning "making fat" literally).

Some of these new fats are retained in the liver, but most of them are transported to other fat deposits in the body. Although this is a more complex procedure, the amount of fat that can be produced is almost infinite.

There are also two complementary food storage mechanisms in our bodies. One is easy to access but with little storage space (glycogen), while the other is harder to access but has almost infinite storage space (body fat).

The cycle goes backward if we don't eat (intermediate fasting). The amount of insulin falls, signaling that the body continues to consume stored energy as food is no longer supplied. Blood glucose is falling, so the body now needs to take off storage glucose to use for energy.

Glycogen is the most open-source of energy. It is divided into glucose molecules that supply energy to the other cells of the body. It will fuel many of the body 's requirements for 24 to 36 hours. After that, the body breaks down fat primarily for energy.

Therefore, the body only exists in two states – the fed state and the fasted state (insulin low). Either we store food energy (stores increasing), or we consume stored energy (stores decreasing). It is one or the other. If food and fasting are balanced, the net weight change should not take place.

Essentially, irregular fasting allows the body to maximize its stored energy. That's what it's for, after all. The critical thing to remember is that it's not accurate. If you eat every third hour, as is often advisable, your body uses the incoming food energy regularly. If any, it does not have to consume a lot of body fat. You can only store fat. Your body can preserve it for a time when nothing can be consumed. As the case may be, you lack balance and intermittent fasting.

Recommendations

As part of an 'intentional approach to food based on timing and duration of meats and snacks,' AHA recommends irregular fasting as a choice for weight loss and calorie control.' Fasting can be incorporated into broader dietary adjustments for over-weight individuals, such as "strategic positioning of snacks before overeating meals," day-long preparation for meals and snacks to regulate hunger better and monitor food quantities, and "consequently encourage fasting overnight." The AHA noted that eating some food on a fast day (rather than a quick day) produced the biggest loss of weight, and insulin resistance decreased when obese patients achieved at least 4 percent weight loss.

The American Diabetes Association "found insufficient evidence of the safety and effects of intermittent fasting on type 1 diabetes" and tentative findings of weight loss for type 2 diabetes, such that no new diabetes strategy was recommended before more study is carried out and then advises that "health services concentrate on the main factors which are common among the patterns.

The New Zealand Health Ministry believes intermittent fasting can be recommended to certain people, excluding people with diabetes, by doctors who note that such "dies may be as effective as other energy-restricted diets and might be easier to adhere to" but that there may be potential side effects during fasting days, such as "hunger, low strength, lightheadedness and impaired mental functioning" and note that healthy foods must be chosen on non-fast days.

The NIA indicated that, while intermittent fasting showed success in weight loss studies on obese or overweight individuals, intermittent fasting in the case of non-overweight individuals was not recommended because of uncertainties about its effectiveness and health, particularly for older adults.

According to NHS Choices, people with a 5:2 diet should consult a doctor first because fasting can often be unhealthy. Owing to the lack of benefit and the increased occurrence of diarrhea, intermittent fasting is not recommended by Europe's guidelines.

HOW INTERMITTENT FASTING WORKS FOR WOMEN

Some women who try intermittent fasting have missed their periods, metabolic irregularities and even early menopause. This could work for certain women, of course. But this is why intermittent fasting can be terrible for your objectives also counterproductive.

So long as I can, my dad eats once a day. He wakes up in the morning and drinks black coffee. It's no eggs, no flour, no muffin. Lunch: nothing more. He enjoys a good meal at home for dinner. Perhaps more remarkable is the fact that Dad owns a restaurant! I shrugged it off as a child. Dads do insane things (he didn't play the accordion at least). He was still in good health and still is at 74 years old today.

My mom couldn't be different there. She is at the breakfast table an hour after waking up, does not skip lunch or dinner willingly, and if the time is too long between meals, she snacks herself off. She's the sort of person who holds her car's almonds even because she begins to feel pecky when she's out there.

I'm not going to say how old Mother is, but she's still in perfect shape, too. Years ago, when I began immersing myself in my career in Nutrition and sports research, I started wondering: how can two people who eat so differently be equally healthy? I had no idea back then that my father was decades ahead – a kind of founder of a now super-buzzworthy diet called intermittent fasting.

Intermittent Fasting And Your Wellbeing

Intermittent Fasting (IF) is a long-term practice without food. There are many ways to do this like meal skipping, alternate-day fasting, Eat Stop Food, etc. There is evidence that, when done correctly, IF can contribute to blood glucose regulation, blood lipid control, coronary heart disease risk reduction, body mass weight management, lean weight gaining (or maintaining) weight, cancer risk reduction, etc.

Fasting And Female Hormones

Playing with IF seems small, right in your life's grand scheme of health decisions? Sadly — at least for some women — small decisions seem to have a significant impact. It turns out that your energy intake is exceptionally responsive to hormones that control primary functions such as ovulation.

Hypothalamic-pituitary-gonadal (HPG) axis, in both men and women, is a little like an air traffic controller in the mutual operation of three endocrine glands.

- First, gonadotropin release hormone (GnRH) from the hypothalamus.
- The luteinizing hormone (LH) and follicular stimulating hormone (FSH) are released by the pituitary.
- LH and FSH act on the gonads (such as testes or ovaries).
- In women, the development of estrogens and progesterone is activated, which will release a mature egg (ovulation) and sustain a pregnancy.
- This stimulates testosterone production and sperm production in males.

GnRH pulses must be timed very carefully, or everything can be released because this chain of reactions occurs in a very particular, repetitive cycle in women. GnRH pulses tend to be extremely reactive and can be thrown away by fasting. Even short-term fasting (three days), in certain women, changes hormonal pulses.

Some evidence also suggests that the lack of a single daily meal (while, of course, not an emergency alone) will begin to alarm us and to put up our antennas. Hence, our bodies can respond quickly when energy intake changes. Perhaps this is why some women do well with IF, while others face problems.

Why Does It Affect Female Hormones Than Male?

We 're not quite sure. However, it could have something to do with kisspeptin, a molecule of proteins used by neurons to communicate (and to do essential things). Kisspeptin promotes GnRH development in both sexes, and we know that leptin, insulin and ghrelin are very receptive, controlling and responding to famine and satiety hormones.

Interestingly, female mammals have more kisspeptin than males. More kisspeptin neurons can make the energy balance more sensitive. This may be one explanation of why fasting causes women's kisspeptin output to dip and throw out their GnRH kilter more quickly.

Putting It All Together: The Study

It would be good to find a human study to explain the research I have mentioned here, but as I said, there are no. Instead, we shall look at a recent rat report: intermittent fasting dietary restriction systems adversely affect reproduction in young rats. A report on the hypothalamic-hypophysial-gonadal axis.

Methods

- The subjects included ten normal-sized male and ten female rats.
- Half of the rats were fed whenever they wanted to.
- Only every second day, the other half ate. Throughout the feeding cycle, they removed their food and fasted.

This lasted twelve weeks or about ten years in human life.

Results

Fasting female rats lost 19% of their body weight by the end of 12 weeks. Their blood glucose levels were lower, and their ovaries were reduced. Ultimately, the experiment influenced the hormones of female rats much more than males. While kisspeptin production decreased both in male and female fasting rats, LH in females fell to four times higher than the average level while estradiol was inhibiting GnRH in humans.

The leptin appetite hormone was six times lower than in a rat that is regularly fed. The experiment took just 10-15 days to interrupt its reproductive cycle. In other words, the hormones of female rats, both reproductive and appetite control, are entirely out of hand.

What does that mean to people? It's difficult to say. But based on what we know about the HPG axis, kisspeptin, hormone-to-appetite relationship and women's environmental sensitivities, it is plausible that fasting can have a similarly dramatic effect on human women.

Fertility, Meet Metabolism

You might think: So, what's the big thing if kisspeptin drops off and I miss out on a couple of periods? Anyway, I don't have children anytime soon. That is the thing here. The reproductive system and the metabolism of women are intertwined deeply. If your cycles are missing, you can bet that there are a few hormones – not just those who help you get pregnant.

Take this snapshot. Women usually consume less protein than men. Fasting women would drink even less. To eat less protein means taking fewer amino acids. The activation of estrogen receptors and the synthesizing of insulin-like growth factor (IGF-1) in the liver requires amino acids. The IGF-1 allows the uterine wall to thicken and the reproductive cycle to advance. Low protein diets can, therefore, reduce fertility. And, above all, estrogen is not solely for reproduction. (Not to mention sexytime.) All our bodies have estrogen receptors, even in our hearts, GI and bones. Adjust the balance of estrogen, and you adjust the metabolism of the entire function: memory, moods, digestion, regeneration, nutrient intake, bone formation, etc. First, estrogens modify the peptides in the brainstem that indicate feeling full (cholecystokinin) or hungry (ghrelin). Estrogens also activate neurons in the hypothalamus that inhibit the production of appetite-regulating peptides.

Do something that allows the hormones to fall, and you will experience much hunger – and consume much more –

than you would in normal circumstances. Estrogens are also the most potent metabolic regulators. Yeah, it is narcotics, it is plural. Since estriol, estradiol and estrogen levels are changing over time. Estradiol is the primary factor until menopause. This declines after menopause, while the estrone remains nearly the same.

The exact function of each of these estrogen continues to be unclear. But a decrease in estradiol can lead to an increase in fat capacity. Why? Why? Since fat is used for the production of estradiol. This can partially explain why it is harder for some women to lose weight after menopause. And that could be a cause to think about your reproductive health — even though you don't concentrate on making children.

And why!?!?!? I know, I know — not fair. I know, I know. People look torn, and you fail to get rid of them. Well, perhaps evolutionarily speaking, if you are female, you shouldn't try so hard to get that stomach washboard. Low-energy diets can reduce female fertility. Too lean is a reproductive nuisance. Female bodies are well suited to any energy and fertility challenges. This makes more evolutionary sense when you think about it.

Human women in the mammalian universe are entirely exceptional. Get this: Almost all other animals will interrupt or delay a pregnancy when they have to. Since the middle school health class, you've known this: women can't. Placenta destroys maternal blood vessels in humans, and the fetus is completely regulated. The baby will block the action of insulin to produce more glucose. The fetus can also dilate the blood vessels of the mother by raising the blood pressure to obtain more nutrients.

The baby is determined to survive regardless of the mother's costs. This phenomenon, which scientists compare with that of the host-virus, is known as the 'maternal-fetal conflict.' Once a lady is pregnant, she cannot sweet the fetus to stop growing. The result: fertility can be lethal at the wrong time, as during a famine. It is not surprising that the reproductive pathway is responsive to many metabolic signals.

How Does The Body "Learn"?

OK, so the hormone balance of women is particularly responsive to how much, how many and what we consume. But how do our bodies "learn" when there is little food?

For many years, scientists assumed that the reproduction mechanism was controlled by a women's body fat percentage.

The plan was to get hormones fucked up, and your time will stop if your fat reserve dropped to a certain amount (around 11% might be a fair assumption). Boom: no pregnancy risk. That makes a great deal of sense. If you don't eat much, you're going to lose body fat over time.

However, the case is probably more complicated. After all, the availability of food can change fast. And as you probably know, if you have ever tried to lose weight, body fat takes a long time to fall, even if you eat fewer calories.

In the meantime, women who are not particularly lean may also stop ovulation and lose their time. That's why scientists believe that the overall energy balance is more critical than the body fat figure.

Stressors And Energy Balance

Specifically, women 's negative energy balance may be the result of the hormonal domino effect we spoke about. And it isn't limited to the amount of food eaten. The following can contribute to a negative energy balance:

- Too little food
- Inadequate Nutrition
- Too much exercise
- Too much stress
- Illness, infection, chronic inflammation
- Too little rest and rehabilitation

Heck, and even energy savings can be taken into account if we try to stay warm. Any combination of these stressors may be sufficient to place you in a negatively balanced energy cycle and avoid ovulation: an exercise in a marathon and feeding flu; too many consecutive days in the gym and not enough fruit or vegetables; intermediate fasting and shrinking to pay for the mortgage.

You think, did she just apply to the mortgage payment? You bet. Psychological stress can play a crucial role in destroying our hormonal balance. Our bodies can not say the difference between a concrete danger and the theoretical that our thought and feeling creates. This stress hormone cortisol inhibits the development of our friend

GnRH and suppresses the development of ovaries of estrogen and progesterone.

Meanwhile, during stress, progesterone is converted to cortisol, and more cortisol means less progesterone. This leads to the dominance of estrogen in the HPG axis. There are more issues. You may be 30 percent fat floating. But if your energy balance is negative, especially when you are stressed, reproduction will stop for a long time to come. Nonetheless, that's the idea.

What To Do Now

Based on what we observe, intermittent fasting would possibly impact reproductive health if the body finds it to be a significant stressor. Everything that affects your reproductive health affects your overall fitness and health. Even if you're not planning to have babies.

But intermittent fasting protocols differ, some of which are much more severe than others. And factors such as your age, your nutritional condition, the length of time you spend fasting and your other stresses – including exercise – may also be relevant. So. So. Is fasting? Is fasting for you? I would recommend a conservative approach, considering how much remains unknown. If you want to try It, begin with a gentle procedure and be careful of how things go.

Avoid intermittent fasting if:

- The menstrual cycle ends or becomes abnormal
- You have a sleep disorder
- You experience hair loss
- You are starting to experience dry skin or acne
- You are noticing that you are not quickly recovering from workouts
- Your wounds are slow to heal, or each bug goes around
- Your stress tolerance decreases

Fasting Is Not For Everyone

The fact is, some women should avoid fasting. Don't try IF if:

- You're pregnant
- You've had a history of unordered food
- You're chronically stressed
- You don't have a good sleep

- You're new to Diet and workouts.

So fasting is not a good idea if you start a family. Ditto whether you are under constant stress or not. Your body needs no extra pain, just nurturing. And if you have had trouble with eating in the past, you will probably realize that a fasting protocol can guide you on a path that could create additional problems for you.

Why do you worry about your health? Similar advantages can be accomplished in many ways. If you're new to Diet and exercise, It could look like a magic weight loss bullet. However, you would be much wiser to fix any nutritional issues before you begin fasts experimenting. Make sure you start with a solid nutritional basis first.

What To Do If Fasting Isn't For You

How would you get in shape and lose weight if intermittent fasting is not a viable option for you? It's easy; it's effortless. Learn the necessary nutritional skills. It's by far the best thing you can do for your fitness and wellbeing. Cook and eat food in its entirety. Train daily. Be positive.

Be trustworthy. And if you would like some help, hire a coach.

Intermittent fasting may be frequent. And maybe your girlfriend, wife, husband or even father considers it an excellent help in fitness and health. Yet women are different from men, and our bodies have different requirements. Listen to your voice and your body. And do the best for you.

THE TYPES OF INTERMITTENT FASTING

Think again if you thought fasting was for religious purposes. A new phenomenon called Intermittent Fasting (IF) in weight loss world is evolving into a common trend in health and fitness. During IF, you move between eating and fasting times. This form of food is sometimes identified as 'fasting patterns' or 'fasting cycles.'

There are many successful IF strategies, but all depends on personal preference. "If you want to try It, brace yourself for the best," says registered dietitian Anna Taylor, MS, RD, LD and CDE. Some people find it easy to spend sixteen hours easily and to confine food to only eight hours of the day like 9 am. Taylor describes to 5 pm, while others have trouble and have to shorten their fasting times. If you are in the best shape of your life or trying to reach those fitness and wellbeing goals, you probably have done some Googling to find the best ways to make your dreams real.

And you probably found the intermittent fasting cycle in your search. If you want to lose weight, increase metabolism, increase your stamina, or even want to feel a little less sluggish after walking up to the fourth floor, intermittent fasting will help you get there. But you certainly need to learn a few things before you start. For all, intermittent fasting is special.

The basic principle of intermittent fasting works this way: you eat about anything you want for a particular duration and then attempt to drink everything but water, tea, black coffee and other noncaloric liquids for a certain amount of time.

It sounds very dull, but there are a variety of different kinds of intermittent fasting. Naturally, everybody's special. It is, therefore, critical that you choose a program that best fits your needs, lifestyle and goals. But if you're ready to dive in, here's five different kinds of intermittent fasting that have become more common over the years.

There are so many ways. This can be achieved, and this is awesome. You can find the type that works best in your lifestyle, which increases the chances of success if you're interested in doing this. Seven here:

1. Time-Restricted Fasting

With this sort of IF, you select a daily food window, which will preferably leave for a duration of 14 to 16 hours. "Fasting promotes autophagy, the normal 'cellular housekeeping' cycle where the organism removes debris and other items that are in danger of preventing the protection of mitochondria, which begins with the depletion of liver glycogen," says Shemek. This helps increase the metabolism of fat cells and optimizes the role of insulin, she said.

For example, you can schedule your eating window to function from 9 am to 5 pm. This can work exceptionally well for someone who eats an early dinner with a partner, Kumar says. Then, much of the time it takes to fast is time to sleep. (Technically, you don't have to skip any meals, depending on when the window is set.) But it depends on how flexible you can be. If your schedule also shifts, or if you want to have the flexibility to sometimes go for brunch, go for a late-night or go for a happy hour, there might not be regular fasting times for you.

2. Overnight fasting

This solution is the easiest of all and involves fasting every day for 12 hours. For example, after dinner, choose to stop eating by 7 pm. Start to eat at 7 am. Next morning with coffee. Autophagy always occurs at a 12-hour level, even though you have milder cellular benefits, Shemek says. That is the minimum number of hours of fasting she suggests.

One proof of this method is that implementing it is secure. Also, you don't have to skip meals; if anything, all you do is remove a snack at bedtime (if you eat one). But the benefits of fasting are not maximized by this approach. If you use fasting to lose weight, a smaller fasting window will allow you more time to consume, and that does not enable you to will the calories you use.

3. Eat Stop Eat

In his book Eat Stop Eat: The Shocking Truth This Makes Weight Loss Simple Again, writer Brad Pilon has developed this approach. His strategy differs from that of other plans by stressing versatility. Simply put, he stresses that fasting just takes time off food. You end one or two

24-hour fasts a week and follow a strength training program. "I want you to believe that it never came to pass when your fast is over, and eat responsibly. That's it.

Wisely eating refers to returning to a regular way of eating where you don't binge because you have just fasted, but you also don't consume or consume less than you need. In tandem with routine weight training, occasional fasting is ideal for fat loss, says Pilon. You allow yourself to eat a slightly higher amount of calories in the other 5 to 6 nonfasting days by taking one or two 24-hour fasts during the week. It's safer and more fun, he notes, to finish the week with a calorie deficit without feeling like you're on a diet.

4. Fasting all-day

Here, you eat once a day. Some people eat dinner and not sleep until the next day, Shemek explains. This means that the fasting time is 24 hours. This is distinct from 5:2. Fasting periods are necessarily 24 hours (dinner to dinner or lunch to lunch), while fasting takes 36 hours at 5:2. (For example, you eat dining on Sunday, fast Monday by consuming 500 to 600 calories and breakfast on Tuesday.)

The advantage is that if you eat for the loss of weight, it is very difficult (but not impossible) to consume all calories of a day in one sitting.

The downside is that it is impossible to achieve the optimum processing of all the nutrients the body requires only one meal. This approach is hard to stick to, not to mention. You might get hungry during the dinner, which will lead you to not so great, calorie-dense choices. Think about it: you don't even want broccoli when you're ravenous. Many people also drink excess coffee to cope with their hunger, says Shemek, which can adversely affect your sleep. You will also experience brain fog all day if you don't sleep.

5. Alternate-Day Fasting

People could fast every day, with easily 25 percent of their calorie requirements (approximately 500 calories) and non-fast days being regular eating days. This is a common weight loss approach. In reality, Dr. Varady and colleagues published a small study in Nutrition Journal that alternative fasting was successful in helping obese adults to lose weight.

The side effects (such as hunger) decreased by week two, and after week four, the participants were more comfortable with food. The downside is that the participants said they were never really "complete" during the eight weeks of the experiment, which makes this method difficult to follow.

6. Pick your day of fasting

It is more a pick experience for you. You may have the time-restricted fast every day, or once or twice a week (fast for 16 hours, eat eight, for instance), Shemek says. Sunday could be a regular eating day, and by 8 pm, you will stop eating and then on Monday at noon, you will start eating again. Mostly, a few days a week, it's like skipping breakfast.

HOW TO DO INTERMITTENT FASTING?

There are many ways to fast intermittently. The methods depend on the number of days and the number of calories. As we learned in the previous chapter, intermittent fasting requires abstaining fully or partially from food for a defined duration before food again.

Some studies suggest that this way of eating can provide advantages such as fat loss, increased health and longevity. Proponents suggest a fasting regimen can be managed more effectively than conventional, calorie-controlled diets.

The intermittent fasting experience for each person is individual and different types are appropriate for different people. In this chapter, we discuss research on intermittent fasting behind the most popular types and give tips on how you can maintain this Diet. There are various forms of intermittent fasting, and people prefer different kinds of fasting. Read on to learn about seven ways to manage intermittent fasting.

1. Fast twelve hours a day

The diet rules are understandable. Every day, a person must decide and adhere to a 12-hour fasting period. Some researchers suggest that fasting for 10-16 hours will allow the body to burn its fat reserves into the bloodstream's energy, which releases ketones. This will encourage weight loss.

The intermittent fasting program of this sort may be the right choice for beginners. This is because the fasting window is relatively small, a lot of fasting takes place during sleep, and a person can eat the same amount of calories every day. The best way to improve the 12-hour is to include sleep in the fast window. For instance, a person may decide to fast between 7 pm, and 7 am. You will have to finish your dinner before 7 pm And wait until 7 o'clock. Eating tea, but would sleep in between for most of the day.

2. Fasting for 16 hours

The 16:8 system or Leangains Diet is called fasting for 16 hours a day, leaving an eating period of 8 hours. Men fast 16 hours a day during the 16:8 Diet, and females fast for 14 hours. This form of intermittent speed can help someone who has tried the 12-hour speed but hasn't seen any benefits.

Usually, people eat dinner at 8 pm and then postpone the next day's breakfast and don't eat again until noon. A mice study found that the feeding period was limited to 8 hours and protected from Obesity, inflammation, diabetes and disease of the liver, while they ate the same amount of calories as mice that they fed whenever they liked.

3. Fasting 2 days a week

Following a 5:2 diet, people consume safe, reasonable food quantities for five days and raising calory consumption for the remaining two days. During the two fasting days, men usually consume 600 calories, while women consume 500 calories.

Typically, during the week, people split their fasting days. They may, for example, fast on a Monday and Thursday and usually eat on the other days. There should be at least one non-fasting day between fasting days.

5:2 Diet study, also identified as the Easy, is minimal. A study of 107 overweight or obese women found that limiting calories two times a week and reducing calories continuously resulted in similar weight loss. The study also found that this Diet reduced insulin levels and improved participant insulin sensitivity.

The research investigated the impact of this fasting in 23 women overweight. Women lost 4.8 percent of their body weight and 8.0 percent of their overall body fat throughout one menstruation period. However, after five days of regular feeding, these measurements returned to normal for most women.

4. Alternate day fasting

There are several variations of the alternative daily schedule involving fasting every other day. One research shows that alternative-day fasting is beneficial for weight loss and heart safety in both healthy and overweight adults. Studies found 32 participants lost a total of 5.2 kg or even more than 11 pounds (lb) over 12 weeks. Alternate day fasting is very severe, and may not be ideal for beginners, or those with other medical conditions. This method of fasting can also be challenging to sustain in the long term.

5. A weekly 24-hour fast

Fasting, known as the Eat-stop-Eat Diet, takes around 1 to 2 days a week, includes not consuming food 24 hours daily. Many people are swift from breakfast to lunch or brunch. Throughout the fasting time, people in this diet plan may have coffee, tea and other calorie-free beverages.

In non-fasting days, people should return to standard eating patterns. Eating this way decreases the total amount of calories consumed by a person but does not limit the different foods consumed by the individual.

A 24-hour fast can be difficult and can cause tiredness, headaches or irritability. Many people consider these effects to be less severe with time as the body adapts to this new eating pattern. People will enjoy trying 12 or 16 hours fasting before transitioning to 24 hours of fasting.

6. Meal Skipping

This intermittent fasting strategy can be perfect for beginners. It also means skipping meals. People may determine which meals to slip through hunger or time restrictions. It is necessary, however, to eat healthy food at every meal.

Meal skipping is possibly the most effective when people track and respond to hunger signals in their bodies. Necessarily, people who use this intermittent fasting method should eat when they're hungry and eat when they aren't. Many people may feel more relaxed than other fasting methods.

7. Warrior Diet

The Warrior Diet's occasional swiftness is a very severe type. Warrior Diet includes consuming very little fresh fruit and vegetables, usually only a few portions, for the fasting of 20 hours, and then consuming a big meal at night. Usually, the food window is just around 4 hours.

This kind of fasting is best for those who have already tried other forms of intermittent fasting. Warrior Diet supporters believe that people are natural nocturnal eaters and that feeding at night helps the body to get nutrients according to its circadian rhythms. People should ensure that they consume plenty of fruit, protein and healthy fats during the 4-hour Diet. There should also be some carbohydrates.

STAGES OF INTERMITTENT FASTING

Intermittent fasting is not just a technique for weight loss or trick that bodybuilders use to lose fat while retaining slender muscle mass rapidly. It is better influenced by human evolution and the study of metabolism in its balanced lifestyle. It demands that the human body be much more effective and self-protective than in modern times.

Many things happen when we easily either don't do it when we 're always fed or when we're in the history of glucose metabolism very slowly. Look down to understand the five intermittent fasting stages!

1) ketosis and extreme ketosis

2) autophagy

3) development of hormones

4) reduction of insulin

5) rejuvenation of immune cells

The cell in your body is in a well-fed state in "growth" mode. The signals for insulin and its mTOR pathways tell the cells to expand, divide and synthesize proteins. By the way, if overactive, these pathways have implications for cancer growth.

"Rapamycin or mTOR mammalian targets have plenty of nutrients, especially carbohydrates and proteins around them. When involved, mTOR tells the cell not to worry about feeding itself, a process of recycling and cleaning (literally, "self-food"), for example, that removes degraded and misplaced proteins. The well-fed cell is not concerned about its productivity and recycling – it develops and divides excessively.

Your cells and their components are also highly acetylated in a well-fed state. That means that different molecules in your cells, including "packaging" proteins known as histones that bundle your DNA nicely into your cell nucleus, are "decorated" in their lysine (amino acid) residues with acetylic groups. Don't worry if you don't grasp the last sentence of jargon. You also need to learn that many genes, including those linked to cell survival and proliferation, are activated for the well-fed cell. Since acetylation typically loosens the packaging proteins that hold your DNA packaged and allows your DNA to be read for protein production.

As your cells activate cell growth and proliferation genes, they also disrupt other genes when you don't fast. These include fat metabolism genes, stress tolerance and damage repair. But things are very different during the famine. When you fly, your body responds to what it considers to be environmental stress (low food supply) by adjusting the expression of genes that are essential to protect you against stress.

We have a well-preserved hunger program that leads our cell to another state when food, mainly glucose or sugar, is not present. If you practice fasting, you trigger the AMPK signaling route. The brake to the mTOR gas pedal is AMPK or 5' AMP-activated protein kinase. AMPK means that the cell is going into a self-protective mode, causing autophagy and fat disintegration. It hampers mTOR. At the same time, the levels of a molecule called NAD+ begin to increase as you do not have the dietary proteins and sugars around which the Krebs cycle typically converts NAD+

into NADH. NAD+, which has Vitamin B3 as its precursor, stimulates Sirtuins, SIRT1 and SIRT3.

(Yes, it became famous as a potential sirtuin activator). (Are you aware of the 'long-term' wine molecule named resveratrol? These sirtuins are proteins that extract acetyl groups we have described above from histones and other proteins. In this cycle, the sirtuins mute the genes associated with the proliferation of cells and trigger proteins to create fresh mitochondria and cleanse reactive oxygen species.

The ketones, which are also produced during fasting, act as inhibitors of deacetylase (that is, holding acetyl groups in place). This enables genes associated with antioxidant processes and repair of damage. Whew, that's a lot while your body doesn't take any calories. But when do these things happen exactly? With a set of LIFE Fasting Arc icons reflecting the five fasting phases, we have helped you imagine the time-line below and in the LIFE Fasting Tracker app!

The Five Stages Of Intermittent Fasting

By 12hours, you joined the metabolism of ketosis. In this condition, your body is breaking down and burning fat. Any of this fat is used to produce ketone bodies by the liver. Ketone bodies or ketones act as an alternate source of energy in other tissue for the brain cells and cells when glucose is not readily accessible. Do you know that when your body rests, your brain uses about 60 percent of your glucose?

When you fast, your liver-generated ketone bodies partially substitute glucose for the brain as well as other organs. This use of the ketone by your brain is one explanation of why fasting is also believed to encourage mental stability and positive mood – ketones generate fewer inflammatory products as they are metabolized than glucose.

You moved to fat burning by 18 hours and produced large ketones. You can now start measuring blood ketone levels above your baseline (for example, 0.6 to 1.0). When their level in your bloodstream increases, ketones can act when hormone-like signaling molecules to help your body increase stress-reduction pathways that, for example, minimize inflammation and repair damaged DNA. Your cells gradually recycle old components within 24 hours and break down proteins associated with Alzheimer's and other diseases. This is a process known as autophagy.

If your cells can not or do not cause autophagy, bad things occur, like neurodegenerative diseases. Autophagy is an essential process in the rejuvenation of cells and tissues – it removes damaged components from the cell, including misfolded proteins. Fasting stimulates the direction of the AMPK signaling and inhibits mTOR activity, which induces autophagy.

However, this only happens naturally when you completely deplete your glucose reserves, and your level of insulin starts to decline. Your growth hormone level is up to 5 times that high when you began fasting for 48 hours lacking calories or minimal calories, carbs or protein.

One explanation is because ketone bodies formed during fasting, for example, in the brain, encourage the secretion of growth hormones. Ghrelin, the appetite hormone, also facilitates the release of the growth hormone. Growth hormone helps maintain lean muscle mass and reduces the accumulation of fat tissue, particularly as we age. It also appears to play a role in the longevity of mammals and can support cardiovascular and wound healing. Your insulin dropped by 54 hours to its lowest level since you started fasting, and your body has become more sensitive to insulin.

Smaller insulin levels have several short- and long-term health benefits. The reduced levels of insulin placed an insulin brake and an mTOR signaling line, triggering autophagy. Reduced levels of insulin can reduce inflammation, make you more sensitive to insulin (and less resistant to insulin, and mainly if your risk is high for diabetes) and protect you against chronic aging diseases, including cancer. Your body breaks off old immune cells and creates new ones by 72 hours.

Long speed decreases the circulating levels of IGF-1 and PKA in specific cell populations. IGF-1 or insulin-derived growth factor 1 is very much like insulin and stimulates development in nearly every body cell. The PI3K-Akt pathway, which promotes cell survival and growth, is activated by the IGF-1. PKA can also trigger the mTOR system (and, of course, there may be too much caffeine to activate PKA rapidly).

You can note that nutritional restriction and fasting will prevent the IGF-1 and PKA brakes, leading to the decomposition and recycling of existing cells and proteins. Researches have proven that extended fasting (over 48 hours) by decreasing IGF-1 and PKA contributes to stress, autonomy and blood cell stem. The same mechanism has demonstrated sustained fasting for 72 hours to maintain healthy numbers of white blood cells or lymphocytes in patients undergoing chemotherapy.

Bonus Phase: Refeeding!

We almost forgot the last stage of intermittent fasting – the refurbishment stage! It is essential to break quickly with a nutritious, healthy meal, which will enhance cell and tissue function when you quickly clean up. Mark Mattson and colleagues at the National Institute for Aging stated: On repair, ingested carbohydrates * and glucose stimulate blood release from enteroendocrine cells of the gypsy hormone glucagon-like peptide 1 (GLP1). GLP1 increases blood glucose clearance by inducing insulin release from the pancreas and enhances cell insulin sensitivity. GLP1 crosses the blood-brain barrier and can function on neurons directly to encourage synaptic plasticity, improve cognition and enhance cell stress resistance.

* Update: This is not a suggestion to break your fast with loads of carbohydrates and sugars that can potentially lead to trouble sugar spikes in your blood. A couple of carbs could go a long way. It's best to break quickly with a balanced meal with plenty of vegetables, plant fibers, plant fats, healthy proteins as well as whole grains or legumes. Stop natural sugars and foods that are processed/packaged. Know what works best for your body and what you feel like to eat after fasts.

And what do you expect? Check the LIFE Fasting Tracker framework for 12-hour, 16-hour, or even 48-hour or longer speed (but speak to your doctor first before long-term fasting)! You will be awarded badges on your fasting arc that provides you with feedback on your progress towards autophagy and cellular renovation!

<u>Glossary</u>

AMPK = protein and cellular energy sensor activated in response to stresses that deplete cellular ATP supplies, including low glucose, hypoxia, and toxin exposure. It causes autophagy. AMPK has been defined as a "key therapeutic objective of treatment of metabolic diseases, including type 2 diabetes and obesity."

Autophagy = a mechanism by which components inside of cells (including proteins) are degraded and recycled. Autophagy can protect the brain cells from the accumulation of "bad" neurodegenerative proteins.

Gene = "basic inheritance physical and functional unit." DNA consists of genes, and specific genes function as instructions for producing molecules known as proteins.

Glucose = primary $C_6H_{12}O_6$ molecular sugar. Glucose is a sub-category of carbohydrates, the most common monosaccharide.

Insulin = "the hormone produced by the pancreas that helps glucose into your blood, which is used as a source of energy in the cells of your muscles, fat and heath." — via NIDDK

Ketone bodies / Ketones = organic compounds made by the liver that are not usable as an energy source for glucose is not present.

mTOR = a protein, recognized initially as yeast, that "controls cell growth and metabolism in response to nutrients, growth factors, cellular energy, and stress." mTOR played a significant part in growth and aging as a central cells growth monitor and has been involved in diseases like cancer, heart disease, obesity and diabetes.

NAD+ = nicotinamide adenine dinucleotide is a cosubstrate of nicotinamide adenine dinucleotide for other enzymes such as sirtuins. "Cellular NAD+ concentrations change during aging," and increased NAD+ concentrations can, for instance, promote longevity through addition.

Sirtuins = anti-aging genes and proteins requiring NAD to function. SIRT1 enables new mitochondria (cell power generating organs) to be produced and harmful reactive oxygen species cleaned.

BENEFITS OF INTERMITTENT FASTING - PHYSIOLOGICAL AND PSYCHOLOGICAL

Intermittent fasting (IF), one of the most widely spoken diets at the moment, means eating and fasting times. And there are no signs that interest is declining. "The IF has a steady pace in its various ways," says Kimberley Rose-Francis, RDN, CDE, a Sebring-based nutritionist. "Actress Jennifer Aniston has recently been quoted saying that It has made a major difference in her life," as stated by Us Weekly.

The two most popular approaches are 16:8, which means you must push all meals of the day into an eight-hour window and fast for the remainder of 16 hours, and 5:2, where five days a week you usually eat and two spend fasting (generally defined as you only eat 500-600 calories a day).

Why does anyone want to eat this way over a regular diet, such as low carbon or low fat? Some claim that fasting has many health benefits. "Research so far has been shown the advantages of IF to the extent that it's worth losing weight, managing your blood sugar and slowing aging," said the author of Hormone Cure, The Hormone Reset Diet, and The Hormone Reset Diet, Sara Gottfried, of Berkeley.

But only a few of them are on board. "From my point of view and the perspective of many others, it tends to fall into the next divine dietary category," explains Elizabeth Lowden, MD, a bariatric endocrinologist at the Delnor Hospital in Illinois Northwestern Medicine Metabolic Health and Surgical Weight Loss Center. Many of the results are contradictory, she notes, and other animal experiments in humans have not yet been replicated. "There are some researches that indicate that there are no improvements for every research that indicates that there is no change," she says.

But instead of taking the arguments at face value, we wanted to immerse ourselves in them and investigate if ten renowned advantages of IF are legit or science is not yet stacked up.

1. Weight Loss

Most people begin to lose weight by IF. And that argument, at least in the short term, seems to hold. According to an article published in the Journal of the Academy of Nutrition and Dietetics in August 2015, a possible contribution can be made by any version of IF to weight loss. Data from 13 trials were analyzed, and the average weight loss ranged from 1.3 percent in a two-week trial for eight weeks.

This may be good news if you hope to lose weight quickly, but since these trials were short-term, it is not clear if It is permanent and will help you keep excess pounds off long. The other fishing is that the amount of weight loss appears to be no more than what you would expect from another calorie-restricted diet, and depending on how many calories you eat every day, you might even gain weight. After all, high-calorie foods are not restricted by a diet.

Dr. Lowden says that when the Diet is appropriately completed IF can be as effective as reasonable caloric restrictions. Some people, particularly busy people who do not have the time to plan meals, may find it easier to follow a time-limited diet than anything like the keto or paleo diet, she says.

2. Reduced Blood Pressure

IF can short-term help to reduce high blood pressure. Research published in June 2018 in Diet and Healthy

Aging showed that the systolic blood pressure of 23 participants was significantly decreased by 16:8. A study published in the European Nutrition Journal in October 2019 found that the IF resulted in even more systematic reductions in blood pressure than another diet, without defined food times.

It is crucial to have healthy blood pressure. High rates can increase the risk of heart disease, stroke and renal disease. Yet work has shown that these advantages of blood pressure only last when It is being exercised. After the Diet came to an end, and people ate, as usual, researchers discovered that blood pressure levels had dropped to an early level.

3. Reduced inflammation

Inflammatory animal studies have shown that IF and overall limitation of calorie can decrease inflammation, but few and far from clinical studies. The authors of a study published in Nutrition Science wanted to know if this connection also existed between humans. The study included 50 participants who fasted the Muslim holiday Ramadan, from sunrise to sunset and ate overnight. The study revealed that there were lower than usual pro-inflammatory markers, including blood pressure, body weight and fat during the fasting phase.

4. Lower Cholesterol

Alternative fasting can contribute to decreasing the total cholesterol and LDL cholesterol when done in combination with stamina, according to a three-week study published in Obesity. LDL cholesterol is the "poor" cholesterol that can raise the risk of heart attack or stroke, according to the Disease Control and Prevention Centres. Obesity researchers have reported that IF decreased the level of triglycerides, which, according to the Mayo Clinic, are fats found in the blood that can result in a stroke, heart attack or heart disease. One warning here: The study was short, so it takes more research to see if the effects of IF on cholesterol last for long periods.

5. Better results for survivors of a stroke

Higher cholesterol and lower blood pressure (two advantages noted above) play a significant role in reducing the risk of stroke. But this is not the only potential advantage of IF connected to strokes. In an article in

Experimental and Translational Stroke Medicine, IF and calorie restriction, in general, is found to have a brain-protecting mechanism. During the case of stroke, the pre-stroke tends to be feeding so that it can avoid brain damage. Future studies are expected to decide whether following IF post-stroke can aid recovery.

6. Boosted Brain Function

Dr. Gottfried says that IF can improve mental acuity and concentration. And the theory has been backed early by research: a February 2018 study of rats published in Experimental Biology and Medicine showed it to be effective in protecting against age loss of memory. According to the Johns Hopkins Health Study, IF you enhance brain function and also protect against amyloid plaques found in Alzheimer's patients. However, this study was only performed in animals, so it remains unclear whether the benefit applies to humans.

7. Cancer Protection

Many studies have shown that, according to the analysis of the studies published at The American Journal of Clinical Nutrition, alternative-day fasting can reduce cancer risk by reducing lymphoma growth, reducing tumor survival and slowing cancer cell propagation. Both animal studies showed the benefit of cancer, and further research is needed to confirm the benefit for humans and understand the mechanism behind these results.

8. Increased Cell Turnover

Gottfried says that an intermittent fasting time improves autophagy, which is "an essential cleaning mechanism in the body for cleaning damaged cells.' Conversely, a break from eating and digestion gives the body a chance to heal and get rid of junk inside cells that can speed up aging, she says.

A May 2019 survey in Nutrients showed that the expression of the LC3A autophagic gene and MTOR protein, which controls cell growth, was increased by time-restricted feeding that researchers described as eating between 8 am and 2 pm. This study was small, and only 11 people took part for four days. Another research, published in Autophagy in August 2019, also noted that food limitation is a well-known way to enhance autophagy, in particular neuronal autophagy, which can give protective brain benefits. Nevertheless, there were also some limitations to this study: This was performed on mice and not on humans.

9. Reduced Insulin Resistance

Gottfried suggests that intermittent fasting can help regulate blood sugar levels in people with diabetes as it resets insulin, although more work is needed. Fasting, such as the fasting of IF, facilitates the reduction of insulin levels that can lead to reducing type 2 risk from the study reports. "I have colleagues in other facilities that have seen good outcomes, in particular in changes to diabetics' insulin needs," said Lowden.

This effect was studied in humans through the Diet mentioned above and Healthy Aging Research. Although a 16:8 approach contributed to insulin resistance decreases, the findings were notably different from the control group. And this study was again low. And again.

Registered dieticians alert diabetes patients to treat intermittent fasting carefully. Individuals with other medications for type 2 or insulin disorder (whether for the treatment of type 2 or type 1 diabetes blood sugar) may be at higher risk for low blood sugar, which can endanger life. Check for any type of diabetes with your doctor before trying intermittent fasting.

10. Lower cardiovascular risk

According to the American Heart Association, the Nutrients research described above indicates the possibility of serious cardiovascular events in patients with type 2 diabetes because they are two to four times more likely to die from cardiovascular disease than adults without diabetes when insulin levels are reduced.

The Nutrients research noted that while no human studies can confirm their utility, observational studies have shown that It can have both cardiovascular and metabolic advantages. Lowden believes that improvements in metabolic parameters, including lower triglyceride levels and decreased blood sugar levels, are the product of weight loss and are done regardless of how weight has been lost, e.g., by IF or a low-carb diet.

11. Increased longevity

Some animal and rodent studies have shown that It could last for longer, perhaps because fasting appears to improve resistance to age-related diseases. In a review published in Current Obesity Reports in June 2019, it is replicable in human studies, although these findings are promising. It is best to be cynical about this possible gain before that happens.

12. A Better Night's Sleep

If you have ever felt like slipping into a coma after a big meal, you know that your diet can have an impact on wakefulness and sleepiness. Some IF followers say that they can sleep better because they practice this way of eating. "IF and mealtimes can affect sleep," says Rose-Francis. Why?

One of the theories is that IF regulates the sleep patterns by circadian rhythm. A regulated circadian rhythm means that you will quickly fall asleep and feel refreshed, although research to support this theory is limited, according to an article published in Nature and Science of Sleep in December 2018.

The other theory focuses on the fact that having your last meal earlier in the night means that you digest the food when you hit the pillow. According to the National Sleep Foundation, digestion is best done when you are upright, and full-stomach sleeper sleep can lead to acid reflux or heartburn, making it difficult to fall asleep.

PROS AND CONS OF INTERMITTENT FASTING

Intermittent fasting is used for a range of diseases over the centuries.1 There are many different IF-styles, from programs that eliminate food on certain days to protocols that restrict food only at certain times of the day. The different dietary patterns received attention as a way of achieving and maintaining a healthy weight and achieving wellness benefits even in healthy people.

Work continues to recognize the benefits and drawbacks of intermittent fasting thoroughly. Long-term studies are not sure whether this style of eating offers lasting benefits.

Pros

1. Easy to follow

Many dietary patterns aim to eat certain foods and limit or avoid other foods. Learning the basic rules of the food style will take a significant amount of time. For starters, there are books about understanding the DASH diet or how to follow a Mediterranean meal plan.

In an eating schedule that involves intermittent fasting, you feed regularly. After you know which intermittent fasting regimen is best for you, it's just a watch or calendar that you need to know when to eat.

2. No Calorie Counting

Not surprisingly, people who seek to achieve or maintain a healthy weight usually tend to avoid calorie counting. No calorie counting. Although food labels can easily be found in many foods, the process of calculating portion sizes and tabulating daily counts can be tedious either manually or on a smartphone app.

A 2011 study showed that when all pre-measured calorie-controlled meals are available, people are more likely to adopt plans.3 Commercial diets such as the WW, Jenny Craig, and others reimburse these services. However, many people do not have the money, especially long-term, to pay for these programs.

Intermittent fasting offers a simple alternative where there is little or no need for calorie counting. Calorie restrictions (and then weight loss) arise in some instances when food is either reduced or substantially restricted on certain days or for certain days of the day.

3. No Macronutrient Limitations

There are standard eating plans that substantially limit certain macronutrients. For instance, many people follow a low-carbon diet to improve or lose weight. For medical or weight loss purposes, other diets follow a low-fat diet.

Each of these schemes requires consumers to adopt a new way of eating – often to replace favorite foods with new and perhaps unknown foods. New cooking skills and shopping and stocking the kitchen may be essential. None of these skills is required when switching on since the target macronutrient spectrum is not accessible, and no macronutrients are limited or prohibited.

4. Unrestricted Eating

Anybody who has ever changed his Diet to make a better health gain or weight understands that he starts to crave things he is told not to consume. Indeed, a 2017 study reported that an increased desire to eat is a crucial factor during a journey of weight loss.

Nevertheless, this assignment is strictly confined to an irregular schedule. Food restriction happens only for those specific hours, and you can eat whatever you want in general on non-fasting hours or days of the program. In reality, these days, researchers often call festivities. Naturally, continued eating unhealthy foods may not be the healthiest way to gain advantages from intermittent fasting. Still, it can cut your total intake off for specific days and eventually provide benefits.

5. Boosts Longevity

Longevity is one of the most frequently reported advantages of intermittent fasting. According to the National Institute on Aging, rodent studies have shown, many of which show an increase in lifespan and decreased incidence of various diseases, particularly cancers, when mice are placed into programs that severely restrict calories (often during fasting periods).

So does this advantage extend to people? It does, according to those who advocate diets. Long-term studies are therefore required to confirm the gain. According to a 2010 review, observational research has linked religious fasting to the long-term benefits of longevity. Still, it was difficult to ascertain whether fasting provided the benefit and whether the associated factors played a role.

6. Promotes weight loss

The authors report that the studies they examined showed a significant decrease in fat mass in intermittent fasting research published in 2018 for subjects participating in clinical studies. They also found that intermittent fasting, irrespective of the body mass index, was sufficient for reducing weight.

However, It may not be more effective than conventional limits on calories. Intermittent fasting may not be more effective than other diets that regularly restrict calories. A research in 2018 compared intermittent fasting to conventional diets (defined as a continuous restriction of energy) and found weight loss benefits to be comparable.

In a major meta-analysis published in 2018, researchers examined the findings of 11 trials lasting 8–24 weeks. The authors of the study conclude that the target was both intermittent fasting and continuous energy restriction, with comparable results. They stated that long-term studies are necessary to draw definitive conclusions.

The effects of weight loss will also depend on age. A 2018 study in Nutrition examined the effects of intermittent (time-restricted) feeding on young (20-year-old) compared to old (50-year-old) people. Intermittent fasting in young men, but not older men, significantly decreased body mass. Nevertheless, in both classes, muscle strength remained the same.

7. Glucose control

Some intermittent fasting researchers suggest in 2018 that this style of eating can help people with type 2 diabetes manage blood sugar. However, the results were inconsistent. A 2018 case series demonstrated the utility of fasting to reverse insulin Resistance while preserving blood sugar regulation. In all three cases, insulin therapy could stop patients.

However, another study published in 2019 showed a less positive effect on blood glucose regulation. Researchers performed a 24-month follow-up to a 12-month experiment contrasting intermittent fasting with continuing caloric limitations in people with type two diabetes. These findings were consistent with other results of studies that indicate that, given a variety of dietary intervention, it is not uncommon for blood glucose levels to rise over time in those with type 2 diabetes. They found that rates of HbA1c have risen both in constant and intermittent calory limitations at 24 months. But the study authors note that intermittent energy limitation may be better than continuous energy restriction to maintain lower rates of HbA1c, but note that further studies are required to validate the advantage.

Other Health Benefits

Some studies have linked transient fasting with several other health benefits. Nearly every study author states, however, that further work is required to understand the benefits better.

For example, a 2018 study found that intermittent fasting during Ramadan reduced total cholesterol, LDL, triglycerides in participants in the study. Another research conducted in 2014 revealed that intermittent fasting (specifically time-restrictive feeding) could be a useful technique for combating low-grade systemic inflammation and some age-related chronic diseases linked to immune function without sacrificing physical health.

Cons

1. Side Effects

Research that examines the benefits of intermittent fasting points to specific side effects during the fasting process of the eating program.

For example, when your calories are significantly reduced, it is not unusual to feel moody, exhausted, and headache. This is more likely to occur when food is entirely omitted (for example, when alternating-day fasting is provided) and less likely if the consumption of food is decreased (e.g., at a 5:2 diet when 500 to 600 calories are consumed during fasting days).

2. Reduced physical exercise

The reduction in physical activity can be a significant side effect in intermittent fasting. Most intermittent fasting systems do not provide a physical activity guideline. Not surprisingly, those who follow the programs may have ample exhaustion to struggle to accomplish their every day goals and will adjust their regular workout routines. Further work has been suggested to see how transient fasting can influence the patterns of physical activity.

3. Severe Hunger

Not surprisingly, it is normal for those who encounter extreme hunger at the fasting stage of an IF food program. This hunger can become more severe if others consume traditional dishes and snacks.

4. Medications

Most people take drugs to find that using their food medication helps to relieve those side effects. Indeed, certain medicinal items are expressly recommended to be taken with milk. Taking drugs during fasting can, therefore, be a risk. Anyone taking drugs should speak to their health care provider before beginning an IF regimen to ensure that the fasting process does not affect the effectiveness or side effects of the drug.

5. No Emphasis on healthy eating

Timing is the focus rather than a food option for most intermittent fasting programs. Thus, no foods (including those without proper Nutrition) are avoided, and no right foods are promoted. Therefore, people who observe the Diet don't learn to eat a balanced diet.

If you're doing an occasional short-term weight loss or medical advantage faster plan, you won't possibly learn fundamental healthy eating and cooking skills, like how to cook with healthy oils, how to consume more vegetables, and how to pick whole grains from processed grains.

6. Facilitate Overeating

Meals and meal frequency are not restricted during the "feasting" stage of many intermittent fasting protocols. Consumers then enjoy an ad libitum diet. Sadly, this can promote unnecessary consumption in specific individuals. For example, if you feel hungry after a full day of fasting, you may be overflowing (or consuming the wrong food) on a day when "feasting" is allowed.

7. Long-term Limitations

While the concept of intermittent fasting is not new, much research into the advantages of this diet style is relatively recent. It is also difficult to say if the effects are long-lasting. Besides, experts also conclude that long-term trials are essential to assess whether the food plan is still useful for more than six months.16 For now, consulting with a health professional is the best way to select and start the IF program. Your health-care team can monitor your progress, including health benefits and concerns, to ensure your food is healthy.

HOW INTERMITTENT FASTING AFFECTS YOUR METABOLISM

As we have known in previous chapters that intermittent fasting is an eating pattern involving periods of food restraint (fasting) and normal eating. This eating pattern will help you lose weight, lower your risk of illness and increase your life span. Some experts also say that it is a better way of losing weight than regular calories due to its beneficial impact on metabolism.

1. Intermittent fasting is highly effective for weight loss

Intermittent fasting is a natural, efficient and relatively straightforward approach to fat loss. Studies have shown that intermittent fasting can be just as effective when it comes to weight loss, if not more than traditional calorie restrictions.

Intermittent fasting in 2014 revealed that people could lose 3–8% of their body weight in 3–24 weeks. Besides, a recent study found that intermittent fasting may be a safer path to weight loss in overweight and obese people than very-low-calorie diets. Ironically, metabolism and metabolic wellbeing will also benefit from this eating strategy.

There are various ways to try intermittent fasting. Many people observe the 5:2 Diet, which involves two days of fasting a week. Some people observe alternative-day fasting or 16/8. If you're interested in trying intermittent fasting, this comprehensive guide for beginners will give you more information. Intermittent fasting is an effective method for losing weight. It can also improve your metabolism and your metabolism.

2. Intermittent Fasting Enhances Various Hormones That Consumes Fat

Many fat-burning hormones are chemical compounds that act as messengers. They travel through your body to coordinate complicated functions like metabolism and growth. They also play a relevant role in weight control. Since they have a direct effect on your appetite, the number of calories you consume and the number of fat you store or burn. Intermittent fasting has been associated with increases in fat burning hormone levels. This could make it a useful weight management tool.

- Insulin

Insulin is one of the leading fat metabolism hormones. It asks your body to hold fat and also stops your body from breaking down fat. Chronically elevated insulin levels will make it much more difficult to lose weight. High insulin levels were also associated with diseases such as obesity, diabetes type 2, cardiovascular disease and cancer. Intermittent fasting has proven as effective as calorie-restricted diets to reduce the insulin level. This eating style could potentially reduce the fasting level of insulin by 20-31%.

Human growth hormone Fasting can cause an increase in human growth hormone blood levels, which is an essential hormone in promoting the loss of fat. Some studies have shown that human growth hormone levels can increase in men by as much as five times during fasting.

Increases in human growth hormone blood levels not only help fat burning but also maintain muscle mass and benefit from other effects. However, women do not always experience the same advantages as men, so it is not clear at present whether women are going to experience the same growth hormone increase.

- Norepinephrine

The 'fight or flight' response includes norepinephrine, a stress hormone that promotes alertness and focus. It has several other effects on your body, including the release of fatty acids in your fat cells.

Increases in norepinephrine usually mean that the body will consume higher quantities of fat. Fasting contributes to a rise in urinary norepinephrine. Fasting will reduce insulin levels and raise human growth hormone and norepinephrine blood levels. These improvements will make it easier for you to burn fat and lose weight.

3. Short-term fasting improve your metabolism by up to 14 percent

Most people claim that missing foods can help the body adapt to conserve energy by raising its metabolic rate. It is well known that very long periods without food will cause metabolism to drop. However, studies have shown that fasting will increase your metabolism for short periods rather than slow it down.

One study in 11 healthy men found that an impressive 14 percent increase in metabolism for three days. This rise is expected to be because of the spike in the fat-burning hormone Norepinephrine. Fasting can slightly increase your metabolism for short periods. However, fasting can have the opposite effect for long periods.

4. Intermittent fasting reduces metabolism less than constant calorie reduction

The metabolic rate drops as you lose weight. Part of that is that weight loss causes muscle weakness, and muscle tissue consumes calories every day. Nevertheless, loss of muscle mass alone can not explain the decline in metabolic rate with weight loss.

A severe long-term calorie restriction may cause your metabolic rate to drop as your body is in so-called famine mode (or "adaptive thermogenesis"). This is achieved by your body to conserve resources as natural protection against hunger.

This was dramatically demonstrated in research of people who lost a considerable amount of weight while taking part in the Biggest Loser's TV show. Participants followed a calorie-restricted diet and an intense exercise regime that reduced weight by significant amounts.

The study found that six years later, most of them regained almost all of their weight. Their metabolic levels, however, did not recover and remained around 500 calories lower than you would expect for their body size. Similar findings have been found in other studies examining the impact of calorie restriction on weight loss. The decline in metabolism caused by weight loss can exceed hundreds of calories a day.

This confirms that "Hunger mode" is real and partly can explain why a lot of people lose weight get it back. Because of the short-term effects of fasting on hormones, intermittent fasting may lower the metabolism rate due to the long-term calorie limit.

A small study showed that a loss of weight in an alternative fasting diet over 22 days did not reduce metabolism. However, no consistency work is available currently investigating the long-term impact on metabolic levels of intermittent fasting diets. One small study indicates that intermittent fasting can reduce the drop in weight loss-related metabolic rate. Further work is needed.

5. Intermittent fasting helps you hold on to muscle mass

The muscle mass is a metabolically active tissue that helps maintain a high metabolic rate. This will help you consume more calories, even at ease. Unfortunately, most people lose both fat and muscle while they are weight loss. Intermittent fasting is believed to retain more muscle mass than caloric restriction as it affects fat-burning hormones.

HOW TO GRADUALLY TRANSIT INTO INTERMITTENT FASTING

It's awful, isn't it?

Someone online can finish high on day 2 of her three days of fasting because she isn't hungry. But instead of being inspired, you say, "It's just 10ams, and I'm starving as a ravenous beast already, I won't last the whole day, I can't do this today." "If you're fat adjusted, it's easier to fast," say the experts. But a deficient carb diet takes several weeks, and you don't want to wait too long. Perhaps you haven't tried it, but you have been thinking about it. "Damn, I can't do that." What if the way to get going was calm and confident? And what if your current skills were sufficient?

Here's how:

Instead of seeing it as another daunting mission, make it a self-experiment, you owe it to your wellbeing. Break it down into tiny but quickly done step by step acts that guarantee that you can conclude, analyze and evaluate what you discover. You don't stick to it; you're here to know.

Since you learn by doing, like most people. Isn't that sounding easier?

Before You Get Started

- Speak to your doctor before you begin. Especially if you have some medical condition or medication. If you feel sick, stop.

- Keep it clear. Fasting in this experiment is described as consuming only flat or carbonated water or black coffee or non-sweetened tea.

- Keep it simple. During the feeding time, eat your regular meals. Intermittent fasting works best in my personal experience when paired with a low-carb, high-fat diet of real whole foods. But launching the perfect combination to achieve the best results is not your goal right now.

- For convenience, time (i.e., 7 p.m.) is defined. You must not follow it. You can adjust the times to your schedule.

- Which weekdays? In my experience, it is more convenient to fast on weekdays because they are more structured and have fewer variables. But maybe that isn't true for you. What you are looking for are those days when you say, "Where is the time? I forgot to sleep! I forgot to eat! "

- Slip-ups are all right. Forgive yourself first. You can collect where you left or continue on Day 1. Do the simplest thing to get you back on track. Next ...

Zero In Your Intent

Why should you want to fast intermittently? What's for you in it?

- Weight loss, control of weight. Fasting lowers hormones like insulin, increases HGH and norepinephrine, making body fat stored more available to energy-burning, so you lose weight.
- Stop narcotics relieve symptoms. Fasting helps prevent diabetes, respiratory disease and decreases inflammation.
- Preventing severe disease, lifespan. Studies have shown that fasting can protect you from Alzheimer's and can help you live longer.

Answer Your Worries

What makes you nervous about intermittent fasting that discourages you from fasting?

- Missing breakfast is all right. It's not the most important meal of the day; it's a simple meal, nothing significant. In reality, breakfast is not gaining weight, and breakfast food is not going to fire up your metabolism.
- It's all right to prevent snacks. Snacking won't help you lose weight, because your metabolism doesn't increase. This research explicitly shows that snacking leads to obesity and fatty hepatic diseases.
- Your metabolism is not going to slow down. Fasting increases your metabolism and helps you to keep more muscle while you lose weight.

There's no need to be apprehensive if your health isn't dangerous. Ready? Let's Start ... "This is the greatest temptation just before you succeed." – Chinese Proverb

Day 1, "Don't eat after dinner

Eat all day long; just stop eating after dinner. It is doubtful that after you had dinner at 7 pm, you're still hungry around 8-9 pm. Especially while you're on the sofa, watching tv, or spending time relaxing with your loved ones. And it usually includes popcorn, chips or ice cream.

Tips to help you through the night:

- Have a glass of water or a warm cup of calming herbal tea instead of consuming food.
- Clean your hair. Brush your teeth. The minty taste can help to reduce cravings. It transmits a subliminal message to eat or brush your teeth again for the day. It's just a barrier you can't eat.
- Sleep it off. Sleep it off. It's all right because you had dinner all day long.

Day 2, Delay Breakfast

Good morning! You've only done a 12-hour fast. Your last meal was last night at 7 p.m., and now it is 7 a.m. That's twelve hours. You haven't been fed for half a day. You eat and fast in a combination of 50:50 ... 12 hours of food and 12 hours of fasting. It's a good thing.

Wasn't that difficult, was it? Everything you had to do after dinner was to stop feeding. When you sleep, time flies! But it's early in the morning. You have to get out of the house, or you're going to be late. So you eat as fast as you can or take something to eat in your car. But why?

Today's postpone breakfast. Feed when possible. Use it when possible. Instead, have a soda, coffee or tea. Nothing drastic delays the first meal until it is convenient. Much like when you got to the office or the kids went off to school rather than in the crazy morning rush.

Settle in when you get to work. Check your inbox, check your calendar, plan your day. Before coffee, you don't have to eat or have food as you do all that.

- 10 AM. It's time to have a demanding meal.
- Noon. Time for lunch. You certainly aren't hungry because you eat. It's lunchtime, the clock says, but the body doesn't know that. It's all right to wait until you're starving again.
- 2 pm. Now you're hungry, have a lovely lunch.

Eat Dinner at 7 pm.

Build on your previous steps: don't eat until 10 am after dinner, postpone breakfast.

Day 3: Don't get a tasty snack!

You've only done a 15-hour fast. Last night you had dinner at 7 p.m., avoided eating and missed breakfast until 10 am. Don't eat before dinner after lunch today.

Tips for stopping snacking:

- Dinner is only a few hours ahead. You know that soon you 're going to eat. You just have to wait.
- Waves of hunger. It's temporary; it won't get worse as time passes, it's going to decrease.
- The starvation might not even be real. Perhaps you're thirsty. If this is a snacking afternoon habit. Perhaps you are tired, nervous, depressed, sad, or bored to eat. Instead, drink soda, coffee or tea.
- Stay alert. Keep busy. Do a work, chore, walk or call a mate. It is time to go home to the dinner that awaits you before you know.

Have dinner at 7 pm.

Build on your previous steps: don't eat after dinner, wait until 10 am for breakfast and don't eat between meals.

Day 4, Skip Breakfast

You've done it! You've been fast for 15 hours – and you haven't snacked. You had dinner last night at 7 pm, avoided eating after dinner and postponed breakfast until 10 pm. Skip your breakfast by waiting for another 1 hour. Lunch will be your first meal at 11 a.m.

Repeat your learned skills:

- You have conscientiously eaten when you haven't eaten during another activity.
- While you waited to eat, you stopped eating out of thirst, habit, or feeling, until you felt starving.
- You felt like short-lived starvation. Do the tricks that helped you ride famine waves before you quit.

Have Dinner at 7 pm.

Make sure you follow the steps: don't eat after dinner, miss breakfast, don't snack between dinner and lunch.

Day 5, Repeat!

You've only done a 16-hour fast. You had dinner at 7:00 PM last night, you missed your meal at 11:00 Am and did not have a snack until 7:00 Am. It's an intermittent fasting protocol called Martin Berkhan's 16/8 process. It has a variety of variations. It's common because most of us aren't hungry in the morning, so breakfast is easy to miss.

Your food window is limited to 8 hours (1⁄3 of the day). You have tipped the scale towards a more significant 2/3 hour (16 hours) fasting period. There are therapeutic results. Repeat: miss breakfast, do not eat after a meal, do not consume snacks between lunch and dinner.

WHAT IS BMI (BODY MASS INDEX), WHY IT IS SUBSTANTIAL, HOW TO CALCULATE AND USE BMI

Your body typically stores energy as fat. However, too much or too little body fat, depending on the location of your body, will increase the risk of cancer. You can reliably calculate the body's fat with a dual-energy absorptiometry (or DXA) unit. It is called a DXA scan. A considerably cheaper option is to measure the total body fat by measuring your BMI.

BMI is a valuable population-level health measure. However, when determining your disease risk, the distribution of fat in your body is more important than the number. That is why your waist circumference is considered a better health risk indicator than your BMI. The increased risk for heart disease, type 2 diabetes and cancer is related to increased obesity of the abdomen. The waist circumference tests abdominal obesity.

Body Mass Index (BMI) is a measure of human physical health and is intended to provide a standard metric for the weight measurement compared with height. In particular,

BMI is measured as a height-divided (squared) weight, as shown below. BMI can, therefore, be seen as the weight to height ratio per unit of height.

BMI = kg/m2 or, BMI = Ibs/in2 * 703

The weight condition of a person may be graded as underweight, average, overweight or obese based on the BMI. Some specialists use a weight group for the diagnosis of "extreme obesity" (or "morbid obesity").

It is determined by dividing the weight into kilograms by meters in square meters (m2).

BMI is for adults only, as children and adolescents continue to develop. This makes it tough for young people to set BMI cuts. However, an improvement in the body fat level in adults who avoid rising is usually induced.

You can use an adult BMI calculator if you know your BMI,

- Weight in kilograms (kg)
- Height in centimeters (cm).

- Within the World Health Organization, the BMI will identify you as 'underweights,' 'balanced weights,' 'overweight' or 'obese.' When the BMI's belongs to:
- Below 18.5kg / m2, you are considered to be underweight and potentially malnourished
- 18.5-24.9kg / m2, you are considered to be overweight
- Over 30kg / m2 – you are said to be obese in a safe weight range for young and medium-aged adults
- 25.0% to 29.9kg / m2.

The general health status can be more relevant for older Australians aged over 70 years than being slightly overweight. Some researchers have proposed for older Australians a BMI range of 22–26 kg / m2.

BMI Is Not Always The Best Indicator Of Safety

BMI is used to indicate population risk rates of morbidity (chance of disease) and mortality (death rate). Variations in BMI among adults of a certain age and sex are usually due to body fat, although there are several exceptions to this law. For BMI computing, the amount of body fat would be overestimated:

- Bodybuilders
- Certain high-performance athletes
- Pregnant women.

For BMI calculations, the amount of body fat will be underestimated:

- Elderly
- People with physical disabilities who can't walk may experience a muscle condition.

Besides, BMI is not a reliable measure for individuals with:

- Eating disorders such as anorexia nervosa
- Extreme obesity.

Why Is BMI Not Always The Best Health Measure Of Health?

In general, the more fat you carry, the greater your health risk. BMI can not differentiate between body fathom and muscle mass, however:

- Muscles

Bodybuilders and those with a lot of muscle bulk will have high BMI but not too heavy

- Physical disabilities

People who are physically handicapped and unable to walk may lose their muscles. Their BMI can be slightly smaller, but not necessarily underweight. In such cases, it is necessary to consult a dietitian who can give helpful advice

- Height

BMI does not ultimately vary from height and appears to overestimate and undervalue obesity in younger people. BMI should therefore not be used as a reference for adults who are very short (under 150 cm) or very tall (over 190 cm)

- People of various ethnic backgrounds

Asians and Indians, for instance, have more fat than people from Europe at a given BMI. In these groups, cut-offs in overweight and obesity can also need to be reduced. That is because, in Asian populations, the extreme risk of diabetes and cardiovascular disease starts at a BMI of 23 kg / m2. Some groups, such as Torres Strait Islander and Maori, have the same risks at a higher BMI.

What Is A Safe Children's, BMI Range?

BMI measurements used by adults are not a useful weight indicator by children or teenagers. BMI measurements are perceived differently to children and adolescents from adults and take into account child or adolescent age and sex.

The current children's BMI charts were produced by the US Disease Control and Prevention Centres. They are helpful for overweight and obesity assessment in children over two years of age. You can use a body mass index calculator for children and teenagers to calculate a child's BMI. However, BMI charts should only be used as a guide to indicate when minor improvements in behaviors can be made and when the doctor or dietitian may ask for further support.

Being Overweight Or Underweight Can Affect Your Health

The correlation between being overweight or overweight and the risk of illness is not definitive. Being overweight or underweight can affect your health. Work is ongoing. Statistically, if you are overweight, there is a higher risk of contracting various diseases. For instance, the risk of death rises from 25 to 27 kg / m2 by 20 to 30%, with the BMI rising. With BMI rising above 27 kg / m2, the risk of death is increasing more rapidly (by 60%).

High BMI Risk Of Overweight And Inactive

If you're overweight and inactive, you may develop the following:

- Heart and blood circulation diseases
- Gallbladder diseases
- High blood pressure (hypertension)
- Type 2 diabetes
- Osteoarthritis
- Specific kinds of cancer, like colon and breast cancer
- Depression and other psychological illnesses.

Underweight Risks (Low BMI)

You could be malnourished and thrive while you are underweight (BMI less than 18.5 kg / m3:

- Compromised immune system
- Respiratory disease
- Cardiovascular disorder
- Cancer
- Osteoporosis.

The Waist Circumference Is A Better Health Risk Indicator Than BMI

When assessing health risks in adults, you should pair your BMI ranking with your waist circumference as a disease risk indicator. With fat around your abdomen or a pot belly, you may develop obesity conditions irrespective of your size.

Fat primarily accumulated around hips, and buttocks tend not to have the same risk for health. People often accumulate weight in the waist area in general and thus experience an elevated obesity risk. Studies have shown that a higher incidence of diabetes, obesity, high cholesterol and cardiovascular disease has contributed to the distribution of body fat. The associations between health hazards and body fat distribution are:

- Least risk – slim (slightly distributed fat)
- Moderate risk – overweighted without a bowel
- Moderate to high risk – slender with a bowel pot
- High risk – excess bowel fat overweight.

Waist Circumference And Health Risks

Waist circumference can be used to suggest chronic disease health risk.

For men:

- 94 cm or more – risks increased
- 102 cm or more – substantially increased risk.

For women:

- 80 cm or more – risks increased
- 88 cm or more – risks dramatically increased.

Although genes of a person appear to accumulate fat all over the center, you can still bring this genetic tendency into account and find a solution to it. The risk of abdominal obesity has reduced by being physically fit, abstaining from smoking and eating unsaturated fat rather than saturated fat.

Why Do You Use BMI?

BMI is a simple, inexpensive, and non-invasive body fat substitute measurement. Unlike other approaches, BMI relies solely on height and weight and has access to the right equipment; individuals may consistently assess their BMI and calculate it accurately. Studies have also shown that BMI levels are associated with body fat and potential health risks. Strong BMI predicts morbidity and mortality in the future. BMI is, therefore, an adequate measure to detect obesity and its health risks. Finally, BMI's widespread and prolonged deployment adds to its population usefulness. It has led to greater accessibility of published population data that allows professionals of public health to compare over time, regions and subgroups of people.

How To Calculate BMI

Calculate your BMI by dividing your weight into a square of pounds (lbs) and multiplying it by 703 by your height.

Sample: Weight = 130 lbs, Height = 5'4 "(64")

Calculation: [130 µ (64)2] x 703 = 22,31

BMI = 22,3

Want not to do this? Using the Centers for Disease Control and Prevention (CDC) adult BMI calculator. Children and adolescents (2 – 19 years of age) use the same BMI calculation, but the results are different for age and sex.

HOW TO SWAP JUNK FOODS TO A HEALTHY MEAL

From salty chips to sugar ice cream cones, it can be oh-so-trial to taste junk food. Fortunately, I've come up with 15 alternative healthy junk foods that will make you feel healthy and tasty! Summer is just around the corner, and that means shorts, tank tops, swimming pool parties, and beach days. Whether you're looking for weight loss tips for "bikini" or just trying to stay healthy in the middle of summer, we can help you out with our healthy junk foods. See 15 alternative weight loss snacks below!

When You Crave For Salty Foods

Potato chips and deep-fried fried foods are classic, quick and straightforward to take. And they're great, that's not the case. Chips and fries, however, are very high in fat and starchy carbohydrates, two things that are necessary to maintain a healthy diet. Moreover, they are often deep-fried. Try baking low-carbon vegetables instead. When you choose the oven, it is easy to control the amount of oil and salt you use when adhering to healthier vegetables.

1. Kale Chips In Place Of Potato Chips

Substitute potato chips with kale chips instead of corn chips. The use of greens significantly reduces the chips' fat and nutritional content, yet still offers you this satisfying crunch. In all your favorite flavors, you can also bake your chips, like Classics (oil, salt and pepper), Sea Salt and Vinegar (self-explanatory), Cheesy (vegan casserole or diet yeast) and BBQ (paprika, chili, garlic powder, brown sugar and dry mustard) for starters. To mimic the comfort of each packet, place your healthy chips in tiny baggage for a crisp and salty treat on the go.

2. Baked Veggie Fries in place of French Fries

Forgo crispily fried and veggie fried roasted. The fried vegetables are as crooked as typical French fries, but they're so far safer! Oven flavored vegetables are easy to get from baked carrots, parsnips and candy a range of nutrients. You can also whip up a savory dip that no restaurant chain can compete with when making fries at home. Or mix mayo, chipotle powder, garlic powder, lime juice, chipotle and water with a little oil.

When You Want Sweets

You can get sweets anywhere when you're sweet, making it much harder to avoid them. When you get sweets The bad news is that the sweet counts for sugar, fat and carb are no joke and certainly nobody's buddy trying to lose weight or eat healthily. A simple way to taste sweetness with natural sugars (fruit, baby sweet, maple syrup) without impacting your health is to find wheat-free choices.

3. Yogurt Fruit Pops To Substitute Ice Cream

Stop ice cream, preferring fruity, frozen yogurt, and dark bananas pop with chocolate. The only way you can handle your frozen dessert is not with ice cream. If you have a creamy mood, blend your favorite yogurt with diced fruit and store them for a few hours in the freezer. If you need some chocolate in your life, dip 80% dark chocolate melted bananas and pop them into the freezer. The great thing about making your frozen desserts is that you can control sweetness, and make large batches that remain well in the freezer for months.

4. Power Balls Over Donuts

Stay away from donut shops for bite-free energy. Power balls are incredibly easy to whip in the kitchen. They are packed with protein and have the same sensation as eating bean holes due to their soft texture.

5. Black Bean Brownies To Replace Cakes

Pass cakes and cupcakes instead and enjoy flourless brown beans. It might sound a little strange now, but we dare try to make some this weekend! You see, chocolate is the essential thing about brownies, and you don't even notice the drinks with the right amount of cocoa powder.

6. Substitute Milkshakes For Homemade Smoothies

Race through the hands of homemade milkshakes and smoothies. When you want a thick cold dessert, and you are warm outside, make your choice of good sweet fruits. However, if you want a balanced smoothie that tastes more like a regular dairy shake, our Peanut Butter Oat Smoothie is filled with a delicious, creamy sweetness of protein and nutrients. Learn how to make your best smoothies here with our free recipe book:

7. Chocolate-Dipped Nut Instead Of Candy

Instead of eating sweets, combine with chocolate-dipped nuts or fruits. The main draw of sweets is the texture and taste mix. When you dip your fruit into homemade chocolate, you can receive the tastes and consistencies that you want while leaving out all the artificial additives that you pour into every commercial candy.

If you want a snap, dip in the freezer and allow it to harden your favorite nuts (you can still dip halfway to minimize calories! If you love chewy sweets, use grapes or other dried fruit. If the freezer can not wait to work its magic, simply dip your warm chocolate into fresh fruit and call it a day.

8. Fruity Sparkling Water Instead Of Soda

Say goodbye to soda and hello to sparkling fruit waters. If you're drinking usual or medicinal sodas, they all have non-body-good chemicals and dyes. To make a fizzy drink cold, slightly crush and mix the fresh fruit in sparkling water or squeeze into fruit juice for a distinct sweet beverage.

When You're Craving Fast Food

Fast food is also the first thing to note when you are stressed and want a quick and tasty meal. Unfortunately, gathering fried or starch food is never safe and does not enable you to fall short. When making home-made versions, you can save the deep freezer and use far less oil, sodium and sugar. The best thing is that there are several fast recipes in a jiffy.

9. Substitute Pizza Delivery For Crust-Free Pizza

Make a crust-free pizza to substitute pizza delivery. You can also taste all the sauce and spicy goodness of pizza without carbs.

10. Bunless Burgers Instead Of Conventional Burgers

Decide to make your lean and green burgers. Lean meat (turkey, chicken, salmon or veggie patty can be used efficiently, and any cheese for the burger can be cleansed from the heart-healthy burger. Buns are swapped into salads, portobellos, or sweet potatoes to make carbs.

11. Baked Chicken Wings Instead Of Fried Chicken Wings

Get your fried chicken fixed with healthy tenders or falafel. Go for oven-backed Panko-Crusted Chicken Tenders, which are fast, delicious and often delicious without the high-fat content of fried foods! Baking falafel is also a perfect way to go if you feel nervous about a delicious meal. Chicken wings are also vital food to kick and watch a game, but they are not very kind to the waistline.

12. Enjoy Burritos Bowls Without Tortilla Instead Of Burritos.

You can easily adjust the amount of cheese and sour cream you use with a Chicken Burrito Bowl. A brand of Paleo has about 200 fewer calories as it does not use milk and maize. A vegetarian version also reduces calories by replacing meat with a heartbeat.

When You're Craving Creamy

Often you want crispy and savory junk food, and it's difficult to find any healthy foods that are low in fat.

Fortunately, without ruining your diet, there are ways to relax.

13. Healthy Dips Instead Of Full-Fat Dips

Substitute fattening dips for healthier sauces instead of full-fat dips. Dips are frequent in chips, crackers and veggies, and this is a great idea we admit. But rather than getting savory cream or cheese dips on the table, pick tzatziki or even a fresh mango sauce. Now that you have a list of healthy junk food choices, you can get to a fit summer without losing fun.

MINIMAL CALORIE DAY FOOD CHOICES

The thought of rising calories every day undoubtedly brings back bad memories for people who have followed a low-calorie diet in the past. The majority of diets include some sort of calorie reduction: some incorporate foods that fill you faster but contain fewer calories, for instance, fruits and vegetables, instead of processed foods. Many diets limit your choices, and eating the same food sources is tedious and less critical.

Other diets combine both strategies like diets that recommend low-calorie foods for most or all of your foods, for example, a tomato, or a particular shake. Recent research demonstrates, however, that low-calorie diets can make a shocking difference overweight.

What Is A Diet Of Low Calories?

A low-calorie diet restricts the intake of men to 1,200 to 1,600 calories per day, and women to 1,000 to 1,200 calories per day. Some people use a very low-calorie diet, often consuming only 800 calories a day for rapid weight loss. This form of diet typically involves individual items such as shakes, bars or soups that substitute food and add vitamins. Very low-calorie diets can aid an individual to lose weight up to 3 to 5 pounds a week.

Most people should consider a low-calorie diet instead of a deficient calorie diet as a means of losing weight. Less extreme diets are more comfortable to follow, less risky and less risky when you are over 50 or have other health problems. Also, gallstones in people who have deficient calorie diets have been identified. Keep in mind that most diets work when you choose healthy lifestyles simultaneously, including increased daily exercise and reduced sedentary time all day long.

Good Reasons For Following A Low-Calorie Diet

The main reason for lowering calories is to help in weight loss. Why else give up anything you like? However, fascinating results from animal research in the animal realm suggest more calorie reduction effects. According to studies in Molecular aspects of medicine in June 2011, it is clear that animals subject to calorie limitation periods, including primates, are:

- Longer life
- Higher levels of physical activity
- Lower rates of cancer
- Less age-related brain degeneration
- Better reproductive performance.

Keep in mind that animal studies and observations involve regular calorie limitation periods followed by or in connection with a healthy diet. In other words, over a long period, the bodies of the animals had time to adapt healthily to significantly less caloric intake.

When People Limit Calories, What Happens?

When I talk to patients about cutting heart health calories, I don't think anybody told me that they wanted to do so to live longer, to feel better, and to have a better quality of life. Yet most people think about how they feel the first few days or weeks after they begin, rather than taking a long-term perspective.

Research published in JAMA Internal Medicine in June 2016 offered a rare insight into how people limit their calories. This study was conducted by people who were not specifically obese since weight loss is frequently used to improve their quality of life and lower risk for diabetes, high blood pressure, sleep apnea and coronary artery disease in obese people.

For two years, 218 participants were followed by researchers in this study. The average age was 38 years, and 70% was female. Up to 28 could have the body mass index (BMI) at the time of registration, but not less than 22. The groups were randomized either to follow their daily diet or to engage in a calorie-limited diet. The diet contained around 25% fewer calories than previously consumed.

Why did the researchers want to reduce calories by 25 percent? They assumed that this amount could be the most reduced and sustained for the entire two-year analysis. Participants worked in groups and had online tools to support their diet. Registered dietitians tracked the participants' weekly food diaries for total calories. All participants were motivated at least five days a week to exercise 30 minutes at a time. The authors mentioned some critical findings.

First and not too shockingly, weight loss for those in the category who ate fewer calories. On average, in this group, people lost 7.6 kg (16.7 lbs) in comparison to people in the other group who lost 0.4 kg (0.9 lbs).

The effect of calorie restrictions on the quality of life was even more critical. Those who restricted calories showed better moods and less everyday anxiety, and over the entire study period, their overall health has improved. The calorie-restricted community also reported better sleep and quality. Finally, the calorie-restricted group felt more excitement and sexual desire than the other group.

Is A Diet Of Low Calories Right For You?

If you are overweight or obese, it can be easy to choose. Weight loss is essential in your overall health to decrease the risk of cardiovascular disease, diabetes, sleep apnea, premature joint disease, high blood pressure, and cancer.

However, reducing the risk of such diseases is just part of the possible advantage of calorie reduction. Many other advantages of limiting calories can improve your life and daily function. This new study suggests that if you are in a healthy weight range, a potential advantage of calorie restriction can also be achieved carefully — as long as the BMI is not lower than 22.

Find the experience of the research investigators in this trial and seek to raise the calories by 25%. This is the amount that has been of value, and that was tolerable at the same time so that it can be sustained.

- Keep a detailed record of your food consumption for one to two weeks.
- Use a calorie counter online to help you determine your calorie intake every day.
- Expect to decrease your consumption of calories by 25 percent during the coming month.
- Write a weekly menu that contains a wide range of foods.

One of the best ways to cut calories is to increase your intake of whole fruit and vegetables that are more packed and less rich in calories. Try changing the diet with other people who can provide social reinforcement and accountability and potent ways to boost the chances of success.

When you start to experience an enhanced quality of life, sleep and other advantages, they help to positively reinforce your goals and make the calorie-limited diet a daily habit. With your feeling healthier, more engaged and a balanced diet, you should be able to visit your local cardiologist less.

One of the most challenging facets of weight loss is calorie reduction. Many low-calorie foods will make you hungry and unfulfilled between meals, rendering over-the-counter and delicious. Fortunately, many balanced foods are both calorie-filled and light. Thirteen low-calorie foods fill up unexpectedly.

1. Oats

Oats can be a perfect addition to a balanced diet for weight loss. Not only are they low in calories, but they also have high proteins and fibers that keep you feeling fresh. One 1/2 cup (40 grams) of dry oats contains only 148 calories, yet 5,5 g of protein and 3,8 g of fiber, which can significantly affect your hunger and appetite.

Research in 48 adults found that eating oatmeal increases fullness sensations and decreases appetite and calories at the next meal. Another minor study linked instant and old-fashioned oatmeal to a substantially improved 4-hour appetite regulation compared with ready-to-eat cereals.

2. Greek

Yogurt Greek yogurt is an excellent protein source that helps reduce cravings and weight loss. Although the exact numbers differ between brands and flavors, a portion of Greek yogurt of 2/3 cups (150-grams) typically supplies around 130 calories and 11 grams of protein.

One study of 20 women examined the effect of a snack with high protein yogurt on appetite compared to unhealthy high-fat snacks, such as chocolate or crackers. Not only did women who consumed yogurt feel less hungry, but they also consumed 100 fewer calories at dinner than people who consumed crackers or chocolate. High protein Greek yogurt has helped alleviate hunger and improve feelings of fullness in a further analysis of 15 women compared to snacks with low protein.

3. Soup

While the soup is often rejected as a light and simple side dish, it can be quite satisfying. Some research shows that soups can be filled more than solid foods — even with the same ingredients.

For example, in a study of 12 people, smooth soup slowed down the stomach emptying and was more productive than a solid meal or chunky soup. In the second study in 60 people, the average intake of calories decreased at lunch by 20 percent before meals. Be mindful that creamy soups and chowders can be rich in calories when they are full. Choose a lighter broth or stock soup to reduce calories and optimize completeness.

4. Berries

The berries are filled with vitamins, minerals and antioxidants that can improve your health, including strawberries, blueberries, raspberries and Blackbirds. Its great fiber content also increases weight loss and decreases hunger.

For example, a cup of blueberries provides only 84 calories yet packs 3.6 grams of fiber. Beer is also a significant source of pectin, a form of dietary fiber that has shown a slow emptying of the stomach and a sense of fulfillment in animal and human studies.

This may also help to minimize calorie consumption and further prevent weight loss. One research showed that a snack of 65 calories with berries reduced calorie consumption later in the day compared to a snack with 65 calories.

5. Eggs

Eggs are highly nutrient-dense because their calories are small, but they are rich in a large variety of essential nutrients. There are approximately 72 calories, 6 grams of protein and a broad range of essential vitamins and minerals in a single large egg.

Studies have shown that a portion of eggs will minimize hunger and improve your fullness. A study of 30 women showed more significant feelings of abundance for those who ate breakfast eggs instead of a bagel and consumed 105 fewer calories later that day. Other studies show that a high-protein breakfast can reduce snacks, slow stomach emptying and reduce hunger-related hormones of ghrelin.

6. Popcorn

Popcorn is one of the most filling low-calorie snacks thanks to its high fiber content. Although there are just 31 calories per cup (8 grams) of airborne popcorn, it has 1.2 grams of nutritional fiber — up to 5% of your everyday fiber requirements.

Fiber not only slows the digestive cycle, but it also stabilizes blood sugar to reduce hunger and cravings. Moreover, popcorn can help reduce hunger and boost your mood more than many other popular snack foods.

In reality, a 35-person study found that those who ate 100 calories of popcorn were more fulfilled and happier than those who ate 150 calories of potato chips. Bear in mind, however, that the benefits are for airborne popcorn. Many prepared varieties have many unhealthy fats, flavorings and salt and sugar added to it.

7. Chia Seeds

Chia Seeds are commonly praised as a severe superfood and are packed into a low calory number with large quantities of protein and fiber. Chia seeds contain 137 calories, 4.4 grams of protein and 10.6 grams of fiber with a 1-ounce (28-gram) portion.

Chia seeds are exceptionally high in soluble fiber, a form of fiber that absorbs liquid and swells in your stomach to promote feeling whole. Indeed, some research has found that chia seeds can absorb their weight 10-12 times in water and gradually pass through your digestive tract to retain their maximum sensation.

Serve or two of chia seeds can be added to your daily diet, which can reduce cravings and appetite. In a study in 24 adults, those with additional chia seeds for yogurt showed lower hunger, lower appetite for sugary food and increased fullness in comparison with the control group.

8. Fish

Fish is rich in protein and cardiovascular fats. For instance, a 3-ounce portion (85-gram) of cod supplies more than 15 grams of protein and less than 70 calories. Some research suggests that increasing the intake of protein can reduce appetite and reduce ghrelin, the hunger-inducing hormone.

Moreover, fish protein can be especially helpful in reducing hunger and appetite. One study evaluating the effects of beef, chicken and fish protein found the most significant impact on the sensation of fullness of fish protein. To further minimize calorie intake, substitute maize fish such as cod, flounder, halibut, or sole for higher caloric alternatives such as salmon, sardines and mackerel.

9. Cottage Cheese

The cottage is an excellent source of protein for those who want to lose weight and an excellent snack. One cup (226 g) of low-fat cottage cheese contains approximately 28 g of protein and only 163 calories. Multiple studies show that increased intake of protein from foods such as cottage cheese can lower appetite and hunger.

Some research also suggests that eating protein can slow your stomach's emptying to prolong feelings of fullness. Besides, a study found that cottage cheese and eggs had identical fullness outcomes in 30 stable adults.

10. Potatoes

Potatoes, due to their relation to fatty fries and potatoes, are usually criticized as unhealthy and harmful. The reality, however, is that potatoes are a nutritious and filling part of a balanced diet. A medium baked skin potato contains 161 calories, but also 4 grams of protein and fiber each.

Indeed, a report measuring the satiety — or fullness — effect of such foods listed boiled potatoes as the most filler, with a cumulative score of 323 on the satiety index — almost seven times higher than croissants. Animal and human studies have shown that potato filling effects can include potato protease inhibitors, compounds that can suppress appetite and decrease food intake to improve the overall supply.

11. Lean Meat

Lean meat can reduce hunger and appetite between meals efficiently. Less calorie, yet protein-packed, lean meats include chicken, turkey and low-fat red meat cuts. For example, 4 ounces (112 grams) of chicken breasts have around 185 calories and protein content of 35 grams.

Research shows that an inadequate intake of protein will increase desire and appetite and reduce calorie and desire rates when consuming longer protein. In one study, those who ate a high-protein meal with meat ate 12% less food by weight during dinner than those who ate a high-carbon meal without meat.

12. Legumes

Pulses such as beans, peas and lentils can be amazingly filling due to their high protein and fiber content. One cup of cooked lenses (198 grams) contains approximately 230 calories, 15,6 grams of fiber and nearly 18 grams of protein.

Multiple studies show that legumes have a substantial effect on appetite and hunger. A study of 43 young men showed that a high-protein meal of beans and peas provided more fullness, reduced appetite and hunger than a high-protein meal of veal and pork. Another study review of nine studies indicated 31% more complete after eating legume pulses compared to high-carb pasta and bread meals.

13. Watermelon

The high water content of Watermelon keeps you hydrated and full while providing a limited number of calories. Apart from a variety of relevant micronutrients such as vitamins A and C, one cup of diced melon (152 grams) contains 46 calories.

Eating foods with a low-calorie density; for example, watermelon has proved to be equally useful for fullness and hunger feelings compared to foods with a high-calorie density. Furthermore, foods with lower calorie density are linked to reduced body weight and lower calorie intake. In a study performed by 49 participants, the replacement of oat cookies with an equal amount of fruit calories substantially reduced the intake of calories and body weight.

Eating a broad variety of foods that fill with plenty of protein and fibers will combat cravings and reduce malnutrition to promote weight loss. These low-calorie foods, paired with an active lifestyle and well-rounded diet, can keep you happy all day.

KCAL VS. CALORIE - WHAT IS TRUE?

A calorie is a heat needed to increase the temperature by one degree Celsius of one gram of water. Food calories provide energy in the form of heat to enable our bodies to function. Our bodies store calories and "burn" them as fuel. Many dietarians count calories and try to reduce caloric consumption to lose weight.

If in nutrition, diet, or merely food-speaking consumers, the word 'calorie,' they usually use a casual definition of calorie. But they refer to kilocalories, as shown on food labels. The concept of calorie (cal) or small calorie is the heat needed to increase the water temperature by 1 degree Celcius by 1 gram of water.

The definition of kilocalorie (kcal) is the amount of heat necessary to raise the water temperature by 1 degree Celcius by 1 kilogram of water. A kilocalorie corresponds to 1000 small calories. Kilocalories are often referred to as 'food calories' or simply shortened to 'calories' when it comes to food energy. Another measuring unit for energy quantification is called "joule." A small calorie is equivalent to just less than 4.2 joules. One kilocalorie (kcal) equals around 4.2 kilojoules.

What's A Calorie?

Although the words "calorie" and "kilocalorie" are used interchangeably, their meaning is not equivalent. The USDA describes calories as a measurement of the energy needed to increase the temperature by one degree Celsius of 1 kilogram of water. You think about a kilocalory (kcal) when you use the word calorie. The real calorie is only a tiny calorie, of which 1,000 take a kilocalorie. A kilocalorie is a calculation of the energy produced in the food you consume. (So, if you consumed 2,000 calories a day, you would consume nothing!) If you use the term calorie and talk about food, you refer technically to a kilocalorie. To better grasp the concept of calories, we need to distinguish research from its conference importance.

Simply put, a calorie is a common word – but kilocalorie is the scientifically correct term. A kilocalorie is equivalent to a calorie (note C). For convenience, then, instead of more technically correct kilocalorie, the term calorie is used.

How Does Your Metabolism Burn Calories?

The key reason we use food is that we supply energy that keeps us alive. When you eat and drink, according to the Mayo Clinic, your body turns the calories you ingest into energy. Calories in the food you eat and drink interact with oxygen to release the energy the body needs.

This process of breakdown and conversion, also known as your primary metabolism or your metabolism, goes on 24 hours a day, be it in motion or rest. However, physically active people consume more calories than those who do little to no physical activity.

- Body composition:

More calories are required in people with slightly slimmer muscle mass. Increasing factors affect the metabolism over time: the muscle is stimulated at rest more metabolically, which means it takes more energy than fat.

- Change of age:

Once people have passed their twentieth birthday, they eat about 150 fewer calories per decade, according to the ACE.

Unfortunately, the body retains more fat, and the resulting reduction in energy (calories) is required and utilized when you lose your muscles with age.

- Chronic and acute disease:

An unmanaged chronic disease may alter metabolism and speed up energy consumption reductions.

So, How Many Calories Do I Have To Eat A Day?

Daily energy needs vary from person to person. Your height, weight, age, level of exercise and muscle mass play a role in deciding how many calories your body needs for rest and everyday life. The American Dietary Guidelines 2015-2020 is a general guideline for age, gender, and activity calorie requirement. Older women can range from 1,600 to 2,400 calories per day, and adult men can range from 2,000 to 3,000 calories per day. The bottom end is for inactive adults, while the top end is for more productive adults.

Both male and female adults aged 19 years and up should receive 20 to 35 percent of the fats 'total calory (with no more than 10 percent of the fats' calories and no calories from trans fats), 45 to 65 percent of their total carbohydrate calories and 10 to 35 percent of their total protein calories.

Calories are weighing units, such as a tablespoon or an inch, according to the Cleveland Clinic. A protein-calorie, therefore, provides the same amount of energy as a fat or carbohydrate calorie. The quantity of energy in each calorie "type" is the same, whether it's fat, protein or carbohydrate.

However, the density of fat, protein and carbohydrates varies. There are four calories in one gram of protein, and four calories in one gram of carbohydrate as well. Fats with a gram of fat with nine calories are denser.

Since fat is denser than the protein and carbohydrates, you can find it easier to satiate if you consume fat because of its higher energy density. Instead, with the same amount of calories, you can consume a more significant portion of food rich in protein or carbohydrates.

When choosing foods and their energy density, balance and consideration of your health status are key. An individual with a genetic predisposition to high cholesterol will benefit from a low intake of fat. In contrast, an individual with a family history of diabetes disease may want to pay particular attention to the types and proportion of carbohydrates he or she absorbs. It is worth remembering if you drink alcohol that every gram of alcohol is seven calories — not as much as fat as protein and carbohydrates.

Calorie Counting To Lose Weight

Calorie counting combined with balanced, nutrient-rich food will help you lose weight. Calorie counting does not always have a simple outcome. It enables people to become more conscious of food choices and to monitor food habits. Calorie counting alone is not sufficient for behavior changes that encourage permanent weight loss.

Due to metabolism changes, a person may gain weight for several reasons. The involved processes are more complicated than the consumption of calories exceeding the production.

- Genetics: Genetics can affect how people gain and lose weight and how their bodies respond to macronutrients and metabolize them.
- Energy balance: Taking in more than one expenditure or consuming more energy can lead to

an unintentional increase in weight. The rise in weight can also result from physical inactivity. The US regular diet provided a surplus of calories from processed grains, saturated fats and added sugar. Consistent consumption can lead to weight gain.

- Hormonal shifts: Deficiency or lack of sensitization of hormones can lead to appetite and satiety in the hypothalamus.

- Stress: According to a study conducted in November 2017 in the Scandinavian Journal, stressors including poor sleep and prolonged workdays and working multiple jobs can call for promoting weight gain.

Intentional loss of weight, done in a safe and balanced manner, takes time and effort. Spurring weight loss should be an individual approach that takes long-term longevity into account for the entire person. Quick corrections and diets of a crash should be avoided.

The development of a healthy food plan that takes account of weight loss is different for each individual. However, all macronutrients from the whole and minimally processed foods can form the basis of a healthy diet, while reducing additional sugars, fats and salts. Your food quality has a direct effect on how your body metabolizes and responds to what you have eaten!

Foods labeled 'low calorie' might not always be the best option — since many of them have a large number of additives and fillers to improve the taste of the food to compensate for the decrease in calories. Although keeping in mind the number of calories you consume to make sure that you have a weight loss deficiency, you should always bear in mind that foods you eat should be nutritious and nutrient-rich.

Choosing nutrient-dense foods combined with calories will help you lose weight with an interactive app, such as MyPlate. For instance, nuts are not low-calorie food; however, the research in the December 2016 Journal of Nutrition found out that people who used energy-dense almonds as part of their energy-controlled diets had better lipid profiles as well as lower waist circumferences and fewer body fats.

For others, weight control strategies are useful when you change the proportion of food on the plate and snacks to maximize the overall calories for the day. Ensure that half to 34 of your plate at lunch and dinner includes non-starchy vegetables rounded off with a mix of lean protein, along with starchy vegetables, bananas, legumes, nuts, seeds, and whole grains, is a perfect guideline for balancing your nutrients. Reducing ultra-processed food, including baked goods, deli meats and candy bars, is suitable for overall health and reduces the possibility of getting chronic diet-related diseases.

TIPS TO FIGHT OFF HUNGER DURING THE FASTING PERIOD

Intermittent fasting is one of the easiest ways of regulating calories and losing fat. Intermittent fasting means to those who do not know; you simply pick out a large window every day where you do not consume calories and a little window when you do it. The most popular intermittent fasting model is the 16/8 model, which means a fast sixteen hours and an eight-hour food fan every day.

For example, you can stop eating around 10 pm and don't eat anything until the next day at around 2 pm. This is such a long time! When you adjust to fasting, it's not that bad, but you may still be hungry before the eating window starts. So here are all my favorite ways to stop starvation while fasting!

1. Drink Water

All right, so this one is pretty apparent. If you fast or not, you must remain hydrated but will want to drink much more water if you do intermittent fasting. It is great to drink a large glass of water for your hydration levels and completely free of calories or other fast-breaking nutrients. But it will give you a maximum temporary sensation, which will help you get the bite out of hunger.

Warning: During IF, you probably will have to pee a lot! All this liquid moves through you without food in your stomach.

2. Drink sparkling water

The sparkling water bubbles have an excellent effect on your stomach, making you feel complete, then you are and much fuller than drinking plain water.

Once again, it won't last long, but for temporary relief and hydration, it's great. Also, one of the most challenging parts of fasting is not able to do anything with your mouth and hands! You don't have to overeat that you are used to anything to eat.

Taking sparking water feels a bit like you have something, and mental relaxation will go a long way. My favorite intermittent sparkling waters are La Croix and any pure, null-calorie water (Perrier, Dasani etc.)

3. Drinking black coffee

Drinking black coffee might get used to if, like me, you like milk and sugar coffee. But drinking black makes it easy (1-3 calories should only be a cup of black coffee).

I start my day with about two cups of black coffee just after I wake up. Some people suggest that I drink it a little later because it enables the suppression of appetite. Again, it is good to have something to do with your hands and mouth to have something in your belly because you can't sleep.

4. Try a Ketosis-friendly supplement

The increase in the Ketogenic diet resulted in quite incredible developments in the nutrition and supplement scene. Have you know that you can drink something like Exogenous Ketone Base from Perfect Keto and keep fast and robust:

- Get more energy
- Kickstart the fat-burning ketosis cycle
- And improve mental clarity

5. Drink Hot Bone Broth

This may or may not be allowed depending on the type of fasting regimen you are taking. Because bone broth has calories. A bone broth cup should be roughly 30-50 calories. It's very minimal and has little effect on your overall calorie intake, although it's fully packed with proper nutrients, so most quick plans allow the bone broth to be quick.

If you find it hard to make it into your food slot, a bone mug (you're going to want to add a touch of salt probably) can be heated up and snacked like coffee. It will fill your belly and taste great while it gives you a surprisingly large amount of protein (about 10 g!) and doesn't add to your total calory every day.

Bone broth is pretty expensive, and because of its caloric content, it breaks "technically" quickly, so it is better to save it for days when you struggle. I love those single-serving packs on Amazon Bone Broth because when I need them, I can catch them without opening a whole jug and running the risk.

6. Drink a Diet Drink

This may or may not be accepted depending on the sort of fasting you do, or may not. Some IF advocates explicitly forbid something that may trigger an insulin spike in your body (the hormone that prepares your body to digest food). There is contradictory evidence of this being achieved by artificial sweeteners.

However, for most of us, occasionally, the diet is okay because they don't have calories. In short, a diet of soda is fizzy, delicious and hits you with a blow of caffeine, which can momentarily suppress your appetite.

Warning: There is some evidence that diet sodas will increase your appetite during the day for immediate relief, so use them sparingly.

7. Chew (sugar-free) Gum

Alright, so we've done a lot of things that you are allowed to drink while fasting intermittently. If you're hungry, try zero-calorie, sugar-free gum if you want to chew something. · (There are debates again about whether artificial sweeteners are allowed in different IF types, but the bottom line is that anything without calories is relatively safe) The gradual release of the taste and the chewing action will keep you occupied and quite happy for a while. This is an excellent strategy to get you to the last hour before you begin to sleep.

8. Focus on a Task

Concentrate on a mission that interests you, something you're excited to focus on or something you can chip easily for a while. Anything that needs you to dig deep and challenge your brain can be a bit hard when you're hungry fog, but it's an excellent time to get rid of if you have a work project which isn't difficult but just involves a specific concentration.

9. Go on a walk

You might think you should conserve energy if you're quick far, but my experience with IF tells me something else. I find that my body tends to tap into its energy stores much better when I get up and walk, like walking. Sitting around to feel miserable appears to make matters worse. But if I get out, get fresh air and drive, I usually feel much better and energetic.

10. Be Social

The most significant diversion is socially being around others! Talk to someone you like, whether it's a water-cooler at work, call a friend like I do, bring your dog to the dog's park and speak with some of the people around. Being social makes your mind and body much more focused and alert, and you'll find that your appetite starts to diminish to a certain degree.

11. Work Out

I find fasting much easier on days than on days where I lift weights. I don't work out on days, I have more time to fill, and I'm not as involved. My body seems to have a tougher time accessing the energy reserves I need to get through fasting.

Many people warn you that you are doing your stomach (and frankly, I 'd warn someone too drastic if, for a short time, you have 300-400 + calories to burn), but anaerobic training like lifting weights is ideal for intermittent fasting. You should note that the strength will not go down during and after the workout.

12. Be Patient

If you've tried everything and you just can't keep your mind out of hunger, you can just have to wait. Hunger also comes in waves during fasting. For a minute, you can be starving and thirsty and then totally OK for the next. Perhaps you can just do this with a glass of water and a solid distraction for 15 minutes longer. You may find that starvation fades after 15 minutes.

13. Eat

You should listen to your body and not put yourself in a risky position. The principle of intermittent fasting encourages eating, not miserable. The target is not to hunger. If you're tired, slow, and hungry, you do have to eat something. And that's all right. Most of the IF benefits come from your calorie restraint. If you still hit your calorie target every day, then you will have no problems. The next day, you will try to get your full pace when you feel better.

HOW TO SUCCESSFULLY COMBINE THE KETO DIET WITH INTERMITTENT FASTING

Cutting carbs and fueling the body fat just gathers energy. But if you are someone who has seen success in weight loss using this simplified approach called the ketogenic diet (or short keto), you may want to take things in one step and combine keto with an intermittent fast to get across a plateau or improve your results. Is there something you want to try?

The response is maybe short, but you should be mindful that this hybrid strategy was not tested or proven to work for weight loss. Experts claim that it may be necessary, but a lack of study means that you might want to think twice before you get to this food approach.

Let's think about what a diet is. What are the basics of a ketogenic diet?

In the 1920s, medical researchers initially developed a keto diet to help in the prevention of epileptic seizures in children. According to the Epilepsy Foundation, this version called the "classic" ketogenic diet or the "long-chain triglyceride diet" requires 3-4 grams (g) of fat for each 1 g carbohydrates and protein.

Today, the form of keto that is somewhat different in that it is a high-fat, moderate-protein, and highly low-carb diet. The fat is about 80% of your day's calories, and depending on your personal needs; you are going to consume between 20 and 50 g of net carbon (carbs minus fiber) each day.

A traditional keto diet list includes the use of dipping most carbohydrates, including nutritious foods such as fiber-rich whole grains and most fruits, while giving preference to fats such as avocado, olive oil, grass-fed beef and sometimes bacon.

This food scheme aims to change the body from one that carries glucose (or carbon) to one that relies on fat for energy. This disorder is called ketosis or ketosis.

The keto diet will, without a doubt, lead to a rapid loss of weight in the short term. However, critics point out that long-term (more than two-year) work is incomplete on people who use keto for weight loss.

Also essential to remember, according to a review published in the European Journal of Clinical Nutrition in August 2013, several claims that keto may treat conditions beyond epilepsy — such as cancer, high blood pressure, polycystic ovary syndrome, diabetes and neurological diseases like Alzheimer's disease.

How Does Intermittent Fasting Works?

Intermittent fasting is another approach to dieting where you plan certain times when you don't eat. There are many ways to do intermittent fasting. For example, some people can follow the common 5:2 IF where five days are "natural," and two are "hot" calories (like about 500). Others could not eat for 24 hours. While others can practice time-limited food, such as eating for 8 hours and fasting for 16 hours.

In IF, there is some exciting work on people that appears, including the role that the technique can play in the treatment of obesity and insulin resistance (the hallmark of type 2 diabetes), a study published in Behavioral Sciences in March 2017. However, the writers of that analysis found that "the health effects of IF are not confirmed by high quality," and it is still unclear the IF form should be observed.

Up to now, IF experiments have mostly been carried out (for weight loss or otherwise) in animals, not humans or are short-term.

Why Combining Intermittent Fasting With Keto Has Become Popular For Weight Loss

Doing Keto or It will support weight loss in the short term even though every diet is highly restrictive, so it certainly isn't for all. But how can they be combined? Can there be two more than one? First, in the view of some experts, it makes sense to merge the two methods. The keto diet raises the levels of ketones in the body; ketones are also increased during the duration of fasting. The brain depends less on energy for glucose when it is in a state of metabolic ketosis. Therefore the transition to a rapid (ketogenic) state during the day will eventually become seamless after eating low carbon or ketogenic for a few weeks.

This is a technique that physicians advise patients in the Functional Ketogenics program at Cleveland Clinic. "The introduction of intermittent fasting will take it to the next level," says Logan Kwasnicka of the Clinic, an Ohio trained doctor's assistant at the Cleveland Clinic. The next step will solve a plateau in weight loss as people will consume fewer calories in IF. The progression of a keto diet can also be natural for those who feel saturated eating so much fat (ketosis can also lower appetite) and do not bother to shrink their food window.

Who Should Try An Intermittent Approach To Fasting?

Anyone who spends more than two weeks on keto and – with their health team all right – wishes to add IF. However, the keto diet has become famous for those with prediabetes or diabetes, but "calling on these patients not to eat for quite a long time can be dangerous," Kwasnicka said. It is unlikely that you will have the right candidate in this combined diet plan if you have chronic kidney disease, a history of eating disorders, undergo active cancer treatment, are pregnant or breastfeeding. Only specific diets (keto and IF) for these populations can not be recommended. Check with your medical team.

Also, you don't have to add IF she notes, if you already follow the Keto diet and are happy and content with the way you eat.

The Right Way To Begin An Intermittent Fasting

Keto Diet In Cleveland Clinic, practitioners do not advise individuals to start keto and IF simultaneously. "The body is surprised by switching from glucose as a fuel to ketones, and This is a big change," Kwasnicka said. That's why people would start with keto. After a couple of weeks or months of the diet, they should think IF.

Choosing the right timing is also critical. Kwasnicka gives its patients a pace of 12 to 16 hours. To many men, it is a common habit not to eat 12 hours a day (say overnight from 7 pm to 7 a.m.).

First, consider delaying your breakfast (from an hour to then extending your time), to get your body used to stretch longer without eating, suggests Shemek. When your current eating routine has been changed, reintroduce breakfast earlier in the day and prolong your time at night as eating breakfast not only enhances memory but also increases metabolism and sensitivity to insulin, according to a report published in the American Journal for Physiology Endocrinology Metabolism in August 2018. As for the length of the stay in Keto-IF, she recommends that she make keto-IF only for six months and then turn to a more normal low-carb diet.

A Sample Menu For Keto And Intermittent Fasting

If you've got the green light from your health team and want to try this joint approach, you might wonder what you are going to eat (and when). Your instincts are right: more about the pacing of this diet.

Below is what Shemek says three days on the plan that looks like in a 16-hour fast 8-hour feed pattern when done with time-restricted food. This is not the only way to Go, there are other ways to fasting. For starters, you can also easily do 12 or 14 hours a day.

You will see that snacks are optional in this plan. Be aware that your carbohydrate, protein and fat must remain in ketosis depending on your health. Working with a keto-IF-known registered dietitian will help you decide specific ratios.

Day 1

- 10 pm. Avocado slices of black coffee and scrambled eggs; all mornings water
- 1 p.m. Lunch Broad leafy green salad with two olive oil teaspoons, 3 ounces of grilled salmon
- 3 p.m. 1/4 cup of Macadamia nuts
- 6 p.m. Dinner Chicken leg (with skin), 1/4 cup of wild rice cooked and 2 cups of turkey cooked with olive oil

Day 2

- 10 a.m. Natural hot tea, keto-friendly smoothie, morning coffee
- One p.m.Grilled chicken breast of 1 tbsp, one whole avocado
- 3 p.m. Snack (optional) non-sweetened coconut chips

- 6 p.m. Dinner 3 oz seated tuna made from olive oil
  on Asian coleslaw bed, covered with olive oil
  drizzle and sesame seeds

Day 3

- 10 a.m. Black coffee with chocolate keto chia;
  water every morning
- 1 p.m. Lunch 3 omelets, 1/2 full pepper and 1 cup of
  spinach cooked in 1 tbsp of olive oil, 1/2 topped
  with avocados, 1/2 cup of tomatoes
- 3.00 p.m Olive snack (optional)
- 6 p.m. Big kale salad (3 cups) with 3 oz shrimp and
  2 tbsp of your choice of olive oil and vinegar

There is no research on the health implications of mixing keto and IF, but it is evident that the ketone rates are that when the plans are combined. This could lead to speeding up weight loss, says Dr. D'Agostino. Nevertheless, everybody responds differently, so that might not be true, he says.

Shemek uses both of its customers' keto or IF and keto. "My clients are both prediabetic and overweight, usually.

When you see and hear the way you eat — and monitor your blood sugar levels — you can live on an IF and prepare keto easily. The effectiveness of the integrated strategy increases its dedication, "she says.

One fascinating way to study low-carb IF diets beyond weight loss are for cognitive health. A low-carbon, time-restricted IF could be beneficial for sanitary insulin pathways and allowing your brain to benefit from cleaner-burning [ketone] fuel, which could provide advantages to Alzheimer's disease patients.

Dr. Isaacson offers an eight-hour feed, 16-hour fast for four to five days a week, personally. This technique will also help to reduce your waist's accumulation of fat. "A larger belly [may] mean a smaller brain memory core," he says. More visceral (beef) fat does not include a higher risk of chronic conditions, such as heart and type 2 diabetes, according to an article published in the United Kingdom Journal of Radiology in January 2012.

Are There Any Known Health Risks And Intermittent Fasting?

Concerning long-term risks, 'people with seizure disorders (what keto has been cultivating for treatment) have a ketogenic diet for decades and have excellent health,' says D'Agostino. However, it all depends, like any diet, on what foods you consume. Bacon and the butter-rich keto diet is different from one rich in avocado and olive oil, and poorly designed keto can lead to nutritional shortcomings. Since adding IF will make you too dramatically decrease calories, you can also lose too much weight or slender mass (muscle), if you push the limit to the extreme. He recommends consuming 1 g per kilogram of body weight in protein each day to maintain muscle mass.

The bottom line is the keto diet with intermittent fasting, a restrictive diet that is high in fat, and intermittent fasting reduces the number of hours you consume. There's a lack of research on each diet alone alongside this combined strategy, so what you do, whether you pursue them separately or together, is uncertain.

If you want to offer a go-to diet, they are highly restrictive, so the low carb count and the secluded eating window can be difficult to adhere to. (Even kids adopting keto to help manage epilepsy will have trouble adhering to the plan!) Make sure to contact the healthcare team before agreeing to follow Keto and IF together. Your doctor will help you to decide whether this combination diet plan suits you and then help you change the medication that you use to make your chances of success better.

HOW TO HEAL YOUR BODY WITH INTERMITTENT FASTING?

Intermittent fasting is one of the oldest nutritional practices of humanity. Our former ancestors have been born in a world of uncertainty and scarcity. Food was not always available, and there was regular intermittent fasting. This way of life left a genetic legacy with crucial health and well-being knowledge. Intermittent speed decreases oxidative stress, increases cell repair processes and seems to be a crucial anti-aging and longevity strategy.

In a world where food was to be battled and won, our ancient ancestors existed. No food passed for several days. Often an extensive hunt will get food for days at a time. This was rare. Usually, one or two big meals were enough every few days to nourish our ancestors.

The Benefits Of Food Shortages

Thousands of years of food shortages have led our bodies to build a defensive mechanism for responding to intermittent food shortages and food shortages. Our cell membranes are more responsive to insulin during food shortages. This is particularly important when food is scarce because it ensures that every bit of food is used or stored efficiently.

The body desensitizes the cells to insulin during periods of food excess to prevent stress from the high-calorie intake. It leads to elevated levels of insulin, fat accumulation and oxidative stress and inflammatory conditions in the body. Insulin also increases cell division, a risk factor for the formation of cancer.

Today we have a large amount of food. We can eat practically anytime we want. Most wellness coaches suggest 5-6 meals during the day. This process nevertheless gives an excess signal to the body that inhibits major tissue repair hormones with critical anti-aging effects.

1. Turning to Genetic Repair

Mechanisms Intermediate fasting acts to activate specific mechanisms of genetic repair that increase cellular rejuvenation. This change seems to make it possible for some cells to survive longer in periods of famine. It is less expensive to fix a cell than to separate and create new cells.

This has a beneficial effect on preventing the development and proliferation of cancer cells.

The release of human growth hormone (HGH) stimulates these genetic repair mechanisms. HGH is known to generate physiological metabolism changes to facilitate fat burning and protein sparing. Proteins and amino acids are used to repair tissue collagen that increases muscle, tendon, ligament, and bones' function and strength. HGH also enhances skin quality, decreases wrinkles and cuts and burns more efficiently.

HGH and insulin function opposites. HGH focuses on tissue regeneration, fuel efficiency, and immune function. Insulin is engineered to accumulate strength, cell division and pro-inflammatory immune response. In this game, Insulin is the dominant player. HGH is inhibited if conditions need insulin release (carbohydrate intake).

2. Fasting is a useful healing tool

Intermittent fasting is one of the most effective ways to minimize inflammation, increase immunity and improve tissue cure. This is one of the reasons why many people are nauseated when infected. This innate mechanism is the body's way to rapidly influence us so that we can create the right environment for natural immunity.

Researchers at the Intermountain Medical Center Heart Institute found that men fasted for 24 hours had an improvement in HGH circulation of 2000 percent. People who were screened had a rise of 1300 percent in HGH. Researchers found that fasting individuals decreased their triglycerides dramatically, increased their HDL cholesterol and stabilized their blood sugar.

The best way to start fasting is by giving your body 12 hours each day from dinner to breakfast. This helps the liver to complete the digestion for 4 hours and the detoxifying process for 8 hours. After this is a natural part of life, try to take the fast up to 16-18 hours one day a week. Ultimately, each week you can decide to do full 24-hour fasting.

Incorporating Different Fasting Methods

- Easy fast: Fast with water only for 12 hours during dinner and breakfast. This helps the liver to finish its cycle.

Example: Finish dinner at 7 pm and do not eat until 7 am on the following day.

- Brunch fast: Simple, fast 14-hour water between dinner and breakfast that moves the body into stored muscle glycogen and body fat for fuel.

Example: finish the dinner at 7 p.m.; eat no more before 9 a.m. the next day.

- Cycle Fast: Three days a week, you easily miss breakfast or dinner for 16 hours.

Example: Finish dinner at 7 pm and eat at lunch the next day at about 11 am-12 pm. Do this every week on Monday, Wednesday and Friday.

- Strong fast: Eat every day in a 6 to 8 hour period. You'd eat two meals a day and fast at breakfast or dinner.

Example: It will involve morning fasting and eating from 12 to 7 pm every day or 8 to 3 pm every day, or whatever 6 to 8 hours you want.

- Warrior Fast: Ancient warriors frequently marched during the day and celebrated at night. Consume all food every day in a 3-5 hour dinner period.

- 1 Day Food Fast: 24 hours a week with only drinking water, greens powders and herbal tea.

- 2 p.m. or 3-7 p.m. During this fast, some may have bone broth.

- Method 5:2: Consume two meals a day for five days and two days each week for two days, eat only one meal and let your body have a 24 hour fast.

How Do I Have An Intermittent Fast?

I like to go to my first meal, 18 hours a day, from dinner. During this time, I generally drink 48-60 oz of water and herbal tea in the morning. Often I'm going to make greens in water powder. Currently, between 12–2 p.m., I eat my first meal and finish my last meal between 5–6:30 p.m. I even follow the 5:2 fasting technique where I make two full-day fasts on Sunday and Wednesday, where I eat only one meal on those days.

I also advise my clients to use coconut oil and grass-fed butter or ghee (1 tsp is fine each) to make organic coffee or herbal tea. It produces fatty acids that are easy to use in the digestive system and instantly provide nutrition in the form of ketones. It contributes to stabilizing blood sugar and stress hormones. This is a useful move if someone struggles with hypoglycemia.

I consider 5:2 and an 18-hour fast every day allows me to feel healthy and vigorous. My digestive system, skin health, and immune system are also strengthened. Experience this and see if you can find the correct pace.

TIPS FOR INTERMITTENT FASTING

Have you heard about the most recent diet, the intermittent fast diet?? There's an explanation why so many actors do so, and so so many people have flourished. This diet isn't a diet; it can become a habit if applied correctly. We all know that these eating taboos don't work through dated diets, such as skipping meals. Intermittent fasting doesn't mean you're missing meals, it doesn't mean that you count calories, it doesn't mean you strictly limit what you consume (what an alleviation!) it just means that you want to consume in some days, but make sure you fast during the others times. It is essential to realize that it is not about starvation but rather a particular division of the calories.

It can help lower blood pressure, raise glucose levels or even slow down the aging process by practicing intermittent fasting (yes, that's a thing) and help you consume fewer calories. When we eat food, our insulin is enhanced, and it becomes stored sugar in the liver and produces fat in the liver. When we rapidly decrease our insulin and then burn out stored sugar. So, if you eat consistently, you'll use your body's incoming food as energy so that your body will never burn the body fat you've stored.

Diets can be challenging and time-consuming, they can limit you, and they can be very costly. Fasting, on the other hand, helps simplify your life and is free. It helps you to save time because you need to prepare fewer meals and food everywhere. There are so many great reasons why this diet will begin and become a habit. Of course, it's recommended to talk about it with your doctor first for any significant lifestyle changes! If you are ready to plunge into intermittent fasting, ten tips are available to help you succeed!

1. Find the fasting time for you

Given the intermittent fasting, which is so adaptable to great success, you need to pick a style that suits you well. There are a few directions to execute it. You can choose the 16:8 or 20:4 process. The 16:8 method includes a 16-hour daily fast (remember a great deal during sleep), and then you have an 8-hour window to eat. The 20:4 system consists of a 20-hour fast and 4-hour feeding time. Both of these methods allow you to start and finish them if you like.

You should split easily at noon and eat until 8 pm. However, if breakfast is more relevant to you and you can say no to snacks at night, a window from 10 a.m. to 6 p.m. could be more successful.

Or, a longer fasting time may be selected. This could include the 5:2 process, which means that you eat five days a week, with two days of absolute fasting. The best thing about this diet is that it is so customizable that you can pick whatever you want or that is more convenient for you and get the same results.

2. Gradually start

It is advised to start a new lifestyle or diet, such as intermittent fasting, at a gradual rate. It allows the body to adapt to a smoother transition. When you fast through your usual breakfast until noon, so you don't try to push up your regular breakfast for 1 hour on the first and 2 hours the next day before lunch without food. Some people are willing to go straight into something new and move through the hard times and hunger, but if you don't want success, do it all the time.

3. Ride Out The Hunger Waves

Hunger will not last long. The next time it feels like the hunger surge is overwhelming. Contrary to the assumption, if you are hungry, it will never continue to build up until you feel like you burst. Finally, it will come to a stop, and you will just have to do so. When hunger strikes, hydration is also vital. Your body can respond to dehydration by showing signs of starvation when you need only H20!

4. Drink plenty of water

As described earlier, drinking plenty of water is so necessary for fasting. It allows you to stay hydrated but also lets your stomach feel complete. You can drink the water you like as much as you want. Even try to drink coffee or tea (but make sure that it is black, cream and sugar split your quick) to relieve all your cravings during fasting.

5. Don't binge

This is so important to fast. Do not split easily with binge feeding. Especially at the beginning, it can be tough not to jump on the most significant meal that you can eat when you break the fasting quickly. You can eat so much too fast and also make bad food choices that your body will hate you later.

The easiest thing to do is to prepare nutritious food when breaking your fasting time to feed and eat slowly. Start with a light meal and try a new snack shortly after you're again hungry.

6. Eat healthy meals

This seems like no brain, but make sure that you fuel your body with wholesome meals between non-fast periods. Many research recommends you use a low-carb diet while fasting intermittently to help alleviate hunger while you fast.

When thinking about eating nutritious food, your body feels strong and stimulates your mind to think well. We all know what it feels like to eat a fast meal, but if you satisfy yourself, you develop a sense of brain fog and feel sluggish and unmotivated for the rest of the day.

7. Stay busy

One of the best ways to distract yourself from the feelings of hunger is to stay busy. How many of you, like me, eat when you get bored unnecessarily. This is because you don't have anything that moves your mind, so you think 'oh, I'm hungry' when you might not be actually in reality.

Seek to take up a new hobby to keep busy. It can be as easy to read a book, hear a podcast, or even clean the house. Even better, get your booty going and keep up with a workout. Nothing is better than encouraging a healthier lifestyle than adding at least 30 minutes of exercise into your day, and without realizing that, while you feel well, you are distracted from food. If you find that you cannot stop thinking about food at work, your job will be reassured. Maybe you need a 5-minute mental break and adjust your focus so that the food thoughts do not linger in your mind and keep you off track of the main point here.

8. Journal

This is a very useful and excellent tip report! Track it all right from the start. If you love technology, you can use your computer, but if you are more of an average person like me, enter a newspaper. It is a good idea to keep track of your daily diet during non-fasting hours and also necessary to control your moods during the entire cycle, good and bad. You will see if you are improving in this way.

If you were angry Monday afternoon, it might have been because your body didn't get used to the new fasting you tried, or maybe it was the big bun you ate at lunch. It's impossible to know whether weight loss habits or safe lifestyle journeys occur if you don't chart them. In addition to monitoring moods and food consumption, take plenty of pictures. Finding is the best way to believe. Make sure you take pictures and progress images well before, so you can focus on how you are making progress.

9. Ditch the Unsupportive People

It is essential to tell the right people when trying a new diet or to do something you're excited about. If you have many negative people or know without hand which people have negative thoughts, don't include them on your new voyage in particular. It is so essential for a new diet or lifestyle to have the right support network. You have to be helped, motivated and promoted by people to help you succeed.

10. Giving it a month

Like beginning a new program or mission, it is also the most important thing. The saying "Rome wasn't built in one day" has unbelievable meaning. For a few days, you can't try to fast and expect drastic weight loss quickly. Your body takes time to adapt, and your mind takes time to make something familiar. When you give intermittent fasting, try to give it a month before you decide whether it's for you or not.

SIDE EFFECTS OF INTERMITTENT FASTING FOR WOMEN'S HEALTH

Remember how your mother used to say that breakfast is the biggest meal of each day? Once you think about it, it makes a lot of sense. The word breakfast means "breaking the fast" in the morning because, since last night, you haven't had anything to eat.

You seem to get snappy when we leave the house without a proper meal because your body has relatively low strength. Therefore, breakfast is an essential meal of the day.

Skipping breakfast during intermittent fasting: Yay or Nay?

People who have been intermittently fasting postpone their breakfast until midday and sometimes even later. One has to follow intermittent fasting for 15-18 hours immediately. For the remaining 8-6 hours, the person can eat whatever he wants.

Times of India told Anupama Menon, a food coach and nutritionist, "Breakfast is an important meal of the day. I never missed my breakfast as a kid because it gave me energy for the day." She also said, "Intermittent fasting essentially means skipping your breakfast. Although we can't make it clear that it's wrong, everyone must do what works for his / her body. "The nutritionist also stressed the relevance of looking after the intermittent fasting. When you are on fast for a week or longer, and you feel drained, fatigued, and your digestive system goes haywire, you have to stop fasting 16 hours instead of 14 hours. If you think it doesn't even suit you for 14 hours, you should adjust it to 12 hours. What exactly are the extended fasting hours? It's not just 16 hours of extended fasting. It can vary from 8 to 18 hours, depending on the comfort of a person.

For any diet, sustainability is supercritical. Whether you have extended fasting or breakfast, you have to realize how safe it is. To achieve your goal, you will live long or forever on the road to preserve health benefits. So carefully decide before you get into something.

Why does breakfast matter?

- Helping people think better
- Helping people stay focused more often

In the morning, people are hungry but different from person to person. For women, a word of caution: Anupama Menon also addressed how severe intermittent fasting can adversely affect the menstrual cycle. She says, "Women are not advised to fast for a minute more than 14 hours because they can take longer and raise their risk of anxiety and depression." For men, she recommends fasting for up to 16 hours.

Why Intermittent Fasting Is Different For Women

There is some proof that intermittent fasting might not be as effective for some women as it is for men. One study found that, after three weeks of intermittent fasting, the blood sugar regulation in women decreased, which was not the case in men. There are also several anecdotal accounts of women who have changed their menstrual cycles since intermittent fasting started. Such changes happen due to the sensitivity of female bodies to calorie restriction. If the consumption of calories is low — such as too long or too often from fasting — a small part of the brain is affected called the hypothalamus.

This may interfere with the secretion of the hormone (GnRH), which activates two reproductive hormones, luteinizing hormone (LH) and follicle-stimulating hormone (FSH). If these hormones can not interact with the ovaries, you run the risk of irregular periods, miscarriage, poor bone health and other effects on your body. While no comparable human studies have been performed, the experiments in rats showed that the alternative fasting periods of 3-6 months decreased the ovary and erratic reproductive cycles of female rats. Therefore, the behavior of women with intermittent fasting should be modified, such as shorter fasting periods and fewer fasting days.

Drinks/Food On Fasting Days

Some experts suggest that you can maintain ketosis as long as your carbohydrate intake is below 50 grams a day quickly. Below are some foods and drinks that you can eat when fasting.

- Water. Carbonated or pure water does not contain any calories and keeps you easily hydrated.

- Tea and coffee. They can be eaten mainly without adding sugar, milk or cream. Some people, however, find that adding small quantities of milk or fat can minimize starvation.

- Distilled vinegar of apple cider. Some people consider it easy to drink 1-2 (5-10 ml) teaspoons of apple cider mixed in water to allow them to remain hydrated and easily avoid cravings.

- Good fats. Some people drink coffee with MCT oil, ghee, cocoa oil, or healthy butter. Oil breaks easily, so it won't kill ketosis, so between meals, it will tide you.

- Bone broth. This rich source of nutrients can help to recharge electrolytes lost only in drinking water over long periods.

Note the foods and beverages containing calories, such as bone broth and the aforementioned healthy fats, split the pace technically. However, limited amounts of these high-carbon, moderate-protein foods do not make your body lose ketose.

Weekly Meal Plan

Are you trying to save money on food? Weekly meal plan If so, begin preparing the next couple of days or weeks in advance. It takes a while, but later it will help you save money. Here are ten tips for a start.

1. Create a guide.

Decide what recipes you are going to make for lunch and dinner. Check out our Family Friendly One Week Menu Plan for these ideas. Instead, on this convenient weekly Menu Planner Template, write your menu. You will be less likely to spend money on fast food or convenience food if you have a plan.

2. Plan your meals around selling foods.

Check flyer shops, newspaper ads and online coupon websites. You may be shocked at the good purchases available. Just make sure you buy and prepare for food that you will need so that it doesn't waste.

3. Plan one meatless meal at least a week.

Legumes, eggs, tofu, peanut butter, canned fish and lentils give high taste proteins at a reasonable price. Here are several tasty meatless dishes: Black Bean Couscous Salad, Egg Bhurji and Sweet Chile Tofu Stir-fry.

4. Check your cupboard, fridge and freezer.

See the expiry dates of your foodstuffs and ingredients. What do you have to use? Search for recipes that use these foods and ingredients.

5. Enjoy grain more often.

Grains such as rice, pasta, barley and couscous are cheap and can be used in various recipes. Use them in soups, stews and salads like Chicken Bulgur Salad, for example.

6. Stop recipes that include a specific ingredient.

Some recipes require a special ingredient you might not have. How much is the ingredient? Is it in a small or big package? Can you use it until it goes wrong in other recipes? It may not be worth the cost to buy an ingredient if you only use it once. Leave the ingredient out or try the recipe at home with an ingredient you already have. It is fun to try cooking, and you may be surprised by the finished dish.

7. Search for seasonal recipes. When they're in season, vegetables and fruit are cheaper.

8. Intend to use the remains.

Consider if you should use residues. For Sunday night's dinner, when you prepare roast chicken with rice and vegetables, make a sandwich of chicken for lunch on Monday. Using the bones for chicken soup on Tuesday and throw in leftover vegetables and rice.

9. Make extras.

Don't let waste any big bunch of carrots or celery. Using anything to make an extra-large pot of soup. Build two lasagna batches rather than just one batch when ground beef is available. Serve one batch for dinner and preserve the other batch in meal portions for another time.

10. Be aware of your family's actions.

Motivate your family to communicate their recipes and help them prepare menus. When available, you can search for preferred ingredients and foods.

MEDITERRANEAN DIET 101: A MEAL PLAN AND GUIDE FOR BEGINNERS

The Mediterranean diet is based on traditional foods consumed by people in countries such as Italy and Greece in 1960. Researchers found these individuals to be exceptionally healthy in comparison with Americans and had a low risk of many lifestyle diseases. Several studies have shown that the Mediterranean diet can lead to weight loss and prevent heart attack, stroke, type 2 diabetes and premature death.

There is no perfect way to adopt the Mediterranean diet because there are many Mediterranean countries, and people may have eaten various foods in different places. This chapter explains the dietary pattern usually recommended in studies that suggest that it is safe. Consider all of this as a general guideline, not a stone. The program can be customized to your needs and expectations.

Basics

- Eat berries, fruit, nuts, beans, berries, potatoes, whole grains, pasta, spices, seafood and extra-virgin olive oil.

- Moderate eating: poultry, eggs, cheese and yogurt.

- Just rarely eat red meat.

- Do not consume sugars, added fats, dried meat, refined grains, refined oils and other highly processed foods.

Avoid Such Unhealthy Foods

- Added sugar: coffee, candies, ice cream, table sugar and many more.

- Refined grains: White bread, whole-wheat pasta, etc.

- Trans fats: present in margarine and various food processing.

- Refined oils: Soybean oil, canola oil, cotton grain oil and other refined oils.

- Highly processed food: any kind of foods labeled "low fat" or "diet" or looking like they were made in the factory.

If you want to avoid these unhealthy ingredients, you must read food labels carefully.

Food To Eat

It is controversial exactly what foods belong to the Mediterranean diet, partially because the difference between countries is such. The diet examined in most studies is high in healthy, plant and animal foods. However, it is advised to eat fish and seafood at least twice a week. The Mediterranean lifestyle includes regular physical activity, the sharing of food and life. You should use these organic, untreated Mediterranean foods:

- Fruit: Apples, bananas, oranges, pears, strawberries, dates, figs, melons, etc.
- Nuts And Seeds: Almonds, walnuts, macadamia nuts, hazelnuts, cashew, sunflower seeds, pumpkin seeds, etc.
- Vegetables: tomatoes, broccoli, kale, spinach, onions, cauliflower, carrots and carrots, etc.
- Poultry: chicken, duck, turkey, etc.

- Fish and seafood: Salmon, sardines, trout, tuna, mackerel, shrimp, oysters, clams, lobster, muscles, etc.
- Dairy: Cheese, yogurt, Greek yogurt, etc.
- Herbs and spices: garlic, basil, mint, minting, rosemary, salad, mustard seed, cinnamon, pepper, etc.

Foods with a single ingredient are essential for good health.

What To Drink

Water would be your Mediterranean diet drink. This diet also includes small quantities of red wine — around one glass a day. However, this is entirely voluntary, and anyone with obesity or issues regulating their intake will stop using wine. Coffee and tea are also appropriate, but sugar-sweetened drinks and fruit juices, very high in sugar, should be avoided.

A Mediterranean Sample Menu For one week

The Mediterranean diet is a sample menu for a week. Feel free to change portions and food options according to your specific requirements and preferences.

Monday

- Breakfast: Greek strawberries and oats yogurt.
- Lunch: Whole grain vegetable sandwich.
- Dinner: a tuna salad made of olive oil. A slice of dessert fruit.

Tuesday

- Breakfast: raisin oatmeal.
- Lunch: tuna salad leftover from the night before.
- Dinner: Tomato salad, feta cheese, olives.

Wednesday

- Breakfast: veggie omelet, tomatoes and onions. A fruit slice.
- Lunch: full sandwich grain with cheese and new vegetables.
- Dinner: Lasagna Mediterranean.

Thursday

- Breakfast: sliced yogurt and nuts. Breakfast.
- Lunch: Leftover lasagna from the night before.

- Dinner: Broiled salmon and brown rice and vegetables served.

Friday

- Breakfast: olive oil fried eggs and vegetables.
- Lunch: Greek strawberries yogurt, oats and nuts.
- Dinner: grilled lamb, baked potato and salad.

Saturday

- Breakfast: raisins, nuts and an apple's oatmeal.
- Lunch: Whole grain vegetable sandwich.
- Dinner: Mediterranean wheat pizza topped with cheese, vegetables and olives.

Sunday

- Breakfast: Omelet with vegetables and olives
- Lunch: pizza from the previous night.
- Dinner: grilled chicken, potatoes and vegetables. Dessert fruit.

Calories or macronutrients (protein, fat and carbs) in the Mediterranean diet are not generally counted.

Healthy Mediterranean Snacks

You don't have to eat more than three meals a day for balanced Mediterranean snacks. But if you get hungry between meals, there are plenty of healthy snacks:

- A few nuts.
- A fruit slice.
- Apples or vegetables for children.
- Any fruits or raisins.
- Leftovers from the night before.
- Greek Yogurt.
- Almond butter Apple slices.

How To Follow The Diet In Restaurants

Most restaurant foods are easy to prepare for the Mediterranean diet.

1. Choose your main meal of fish or seafood.

2. Please ask them to fry in extra virgin olive oil your food.

3. Eat just whole grain bread with olive oil rather than butter.

A Quick Shopping List For The Diet

Shopping on the edge of the shop is also a good idea. Usually, that's where the entire food is. Often try selecting the least processed alternative. Bio is the best, but only if you can afford it easily.

- Veggies: Variety of mixtures of organic vegetables such as carrots, onions, broccoli, spinach, kale, garlic, etc.
- Fruit: Apple, Banana, Peach, Grapes, etc.
- Fish: salmon, sardines, trout.
- Grain: Whole-grain Rice, full-grains pasta, etc...
- Legumes: lens, peas, beans, etc.
- Grain: Sunflower seeds, pumpkin seeds, etc...
- Shrimp and crustaceans.
- Sweet potatoes and onions.
- Meat.
- Greek Yogurt.
- Chicken.
- Fortified eggs or omega-3.
- Extra virgin Olive oil.

It is best to clear up all unhealthy temptations, including sodas, ice cream, cookies, pastries, white bread, crackers and fried foods from your house. You can only consume nutritious food if you have good food in your house.

FAQ

Fasting Myths

Men and women of all ages have jumped on this fitness and wellness trend to help them lose weight and improve their health. Once you go ahead in the footsteps of supposed followers, you want to precisely know what this kind of "diet" really means. Although fasting is right for your mind and body, there are also things you should be careful about when you are finished.

"Those who easily enjoy high calorie, high-fat foods with the illusion that fasting helps them to devour whatever they want. The physiological urge to overeat is when you deprive your body of food because of the release of hormones of appetite like ghrelin and leptin and the anticipation of the hunger centers in your brain. Indeed, intermittent fasting, a dietary pattern that runs between fasting and food, is also marketed as a miracle diet. However, not everything you learned about the frequency of meals and your wellbeing is real.

Here are 11 myths on the duration of fasting and food.

1. Skipping breakfast makes you fat.

One enduring misconception is that breakfast is the most important meal of the day. Missing breakfast makes you fat Many also assume that missing breakfast leads to unnecessary starvation, cravings and increased weight. A 16-week study of 283 overweight and obese adults showed no difference in weight between breakfast eats and breakfast eaters.

Breakfast also does not affect your weight to a high degree, although there may be some individual variation. Some studies even suggest that long-term breakfast users tend to lose weight. Moreover, children and adolescents having breakfast continue to do better at school.

As such, it is essential to take care of your unique needs. Breakfast is perfect for some men, while others will miss it without adverse consequences. Many people can benefit from breakfast, but it's not necessary for your safety. Regulated studies indicate no weight loss difference between those who eat breakfast and those who miss breakfast.

2. Frequently eating boosts your metabolism

Many people assume that consuming more food raises the rate of metabolism, which raises the body's daily calories. Your body also uses some calories to digest meals. It is called thermal effect food (TEF).

TEF uses about 10 percent of the calorie intake on average. What counts, though, is the overall number of calories you consume, not how much food you eat. Six five hundred-calorie foods have the same effect as three thousand-calorie foods. With an average TEF of 10%, 300 calories will be burned in both cases.

Many studies show that rising or reducing food frequency does not affect total burned calories. Unlike common opinion, consuming smaller foods does not increase metabolism more often.

3. Frequently eating reduces hunger.

Some people claim that intermittent feeding helps avoid cravings and prolonged starvation. However, the evidence is mixed. Although some studies show that eating more frequent meals leads to less hunger, other studies have found no effect or even hunger.

A study comparing eating three or six high-protein foods a day found that eating three foods decreased famine more effectively. That said, the answers can depend on the individual. If your cravings are that by daily feeding, it is probably a good idea. However, no evidence snacking or feeding reduces everyone's appetite more often.

No convincing proof exists that eating more often decreases the overall intake of hunger or calories. Instead, several studies have shown that smaller, more popular foods increase hunger.

4. Frequent meals can help you lose weight Host meals will help you lose weight Because eating more often doesn't improve your metabolism, it also does not affect weight loss. In 16 adults with obesity, the effects of eating 3 and 6 foods per day were compared, and weight, fat loss or appetite did not differ.

Some people complain that it is always harder for them to adopt a balanced diet to eat. If, however, it is easier for you to eat fewer calories and less junk food, feel free to stick to it. No evidence changing the number of meals helps you lose weight.

5. Your brain needs a regular supply of dietary glucose.

Some people suggest that the brain keeps working if you don't consume carbohydrates every few hours. It is based on the conviction that the brain can use fuel only with glucose. However, the glucose your body requires can easily be generated through a process called gluconeogenesis.

Your body can also generate ketone from dietary fats during long-term fasting, starvation or extremely low-carb diets. Ketone bodies can feed your brain and significantly reduce their glucose requirement.

However, some people report that when they don't eat for a while, they are tired or shaky. If this is true for you, consider snacking or eating more often. Your body can only produce glucose to fuel your brain, which means you do not need a daily dietary intake of glucose.

6. Eating often is right for your health

Some people believe that continuous food improves your body. Eating is also good for your health. In the short term, however, a cell repair procedure called autophagy induces an energy process, in which your cells use old and dysfunctional proteins.

Autophagy can help protect people from aging, cancer and diseases such as Alzheimer's disease. Occasional fasting, therefore, has multiple benefits for your metabolic wellbeing. Some research also shows that eating or snacking also impacts your health and raises the risk of illness.

One research has shown, for example, that a high-calorie diet with several meals dramatically improves liver fat, suggesting an increased risk of fatty liver disease. Furthermore, other observational studies indicate that people eating more regularly have a much higher risk of colorectal cancer. It's a fallacy that snacking is healthy for your wellbeing necessarily. Instead, fasting has significant health benefits from time to time.

7. Fasting puts your body in starvation mode

A common reason against intermittent fasting is that it puts your body in a hunger mode, thereby reducing your metabolism and stopping you from losing fat. Fasting puts your body in a hunger mode. Although, a long-term loss of weight will indeed reduce the number of calories you eat over time, no matter what type of losing weight you use. There is no proof that intermittent fasting contributes to a more significant reduction in burnt calories than other weight loss approaches. Short-term fasting will increase your metabolic rate.

This is because norepinephrine rises significantly in the blood, which enhances your metabolism and instructs your fat cells to break down body fat. Studies show that fasting can increase metabolism by 3.6 to 14 percent for up to 48 hours. However, if you drive a lot longer, the results will shift and your metabolism decrease.

One research found that fasting for 22 days every other day did not lead to a caloric reduction but an average fat weight loss of 4%. Short-term fasting doesn't make the body thirsty. Alternatively, the metabolism improves by up to 48 hours in fasts.

8. Your body can only use a certain amount of protein per meal

Some people say you can only consume 30 grams of protein a meal and should eat every 2–3 hours to optimize muscle production. Your body can only eat a certain amount of protein a day. However, science does not help this. Studies suggest that consuming the protein in more regular levels does not affect muscle mass. The critical difference for certain people is the actual amount of protein consumed — not the amount of food it spreads. Your body can use over 30 grams of protein per meal easily. Protein is excessive every 2–3 hours.

9. Intermittent fasting allows you to lose your muscle

Some people claim that your body burns muscle for fuel when you fast. While this is usually the case for food, no evidence suggests that intermittent fasting is more prevalent than other approaches. On the other hand, studies indicate that intermittent fasting is ideal for mass muscle maintenance. Intermittent fasting in an analysis caused a similar amount of loss of weight as a continuous reduction in calories but with much less muscle mass reduction.

Of another study, people who ate all their calories for a big dinner in the evening reported a small increase in muscle mass. Intermittent fasting is especially common with many bodybuilders who find that it helps preserve their muscles alongside a low percentage of body fat. There is no evidence that fasting causes more loss of muscle than regular calories. Studies show that intermittent fasting can help you maintain muscle mass during your diet.

10. Intermittent fasting is harmful to your health

While you may have heard reports that intermittent fasting is detrimental to your wellbeing, studies show that it provides many remarkable health benefits. For example, it affects the longevity and immunity of your gene expression and has been shown to prolong the life of animals.

It also has significant metabolic health benefits, including higher insulin sensitivity and decreased oxidative stress, inflammation and the risk of heart disease. It can also improve brain wellbeing by boosting the BDNF, a hormone that can protect against depression and many other mental illnesses. While rumors circulate that fasting is dangerous, it has health benefits for your brain and body.

11. Intermittent fasting makes you overeat

Some people claim that intermittent fasting causes you to overcrowd during eating times. While it is true that you can compensate for the calories lost quickly by eating a little later automatically, this compensation is not complete.

One research found that people who fasted only for 24 hours eventually consumed about 500 extra calories the next day, much less than the 2,400 calories they lost during the rap. Since it reduces the overall food intake and the level of insulin while increasing the level of metabolism, norepinephrine and human growth hormone (HGH), you lose fat, not attain it.

According to one study, the average weight and belly fat losses for 3–24 weeks were 3–8% and 4–7%, respectively. Intermittent fasting can, therefore, be one of the most effective methods for weight loss. Intermittent fasting is an essential form of weight loss. No research suggests intermittent fasting encourages weight gain, despite reports to the contrary.

Many myths are perpetuated about the intermittent frequency of fasting and food. Many of these rumors are not true, however. Eating smaller, more regular foods, for example, will not improve or reduce metabolism. Moreover, intermittent fasting is far from dangerous — and may offer many advantages. Before jumping to conclusions about your metabolism and overall health, you may review sources or do a little analysis.

Who Shouldn't Try It

Intermittent fasting seems to be the latest phenomenon among businesses. Intermittent fasting is a fixed time that a person does not eat food intentionally. There are many forms of fasting methods, as there are several different types of diets. From the 12-hour fast to the alternative day fast, many kinds of fasting are becoming ever more common. After intermittent fasting, the body starts to burn fat around 12-24 hours after starving after the body is saturated with carbohydrates, and thus, starving the body of food for 12-24 hours can lead to weight loss that can improve the health.

However, most research on this subject has been carried out over a brief period on animals and has assessed glucose levels instead of long-term health outcomes. Many believe that intermittent fasting is not inherently unhealthy. However, others accept that it is not safe to fast intermittently. So yes, calories, fat and weight may be lost from this typical diet. Still, it is also possible to regain the weight as quickly, to develop low energy reserves, which can lead to depressed mood, sleep difficulties, and even organ damage if the fasting is severe. The following are explanations why people should stop intermittent fasting: Whether you have higher caloric requirements, underweight people, have trouble with weight gain, under 18, are pregnant, or breastfeeding, don't pursue an intermittent fasting diet as they need adequate calories to grow effectively every day.

When you are exposed to an eating disorder, intermittent fasting is strongly correlated with bulimic nervousness, and individuals vulnerable to the eating disorder should, therefore, not undergo any diet correlated with fasting. You should stop fasting entirely. Risk factors include a family member with an eating disorder, perfectionism, impulsiveness and mood instability.

You would most probably feel hungry, overweight, dehydrated and exhausted. Intermittent fasting is not for weariness of the heart, which means that, even though you are not overweight, you are not over 18 years of age, so you are not susceptible to an eating disease.

- You will often experience a rumbling stomach, mainly if you are used to grazing continuously all day long. To stop these pains during fasting times, do not look, smell or even talk about food, which can release gastric acid in your stomach and make you hungry.
- Fast-free days are not days where you can splurge on what you want because that will lead to weight gain. Fasting can also increase cortisol, a stress hormone, which can contribute to even more food cravings. Remember that excessive consumption and binge eating are two typical adverse effects of intermittent fasting.
- Intermittent fasting is often associated with dehydration, as you often forget to be thirsty when

you do not eat. It is, therefore, essential to remain adequately hydrated all day long by drinking, on average, three liters of water.

- You will probably feel exhausted since your body has less strength than usual, and because fasting can increase tension, it can also disrupt your sleep patterns. It is, therefore, essential to follow a safe, routine sleep pattern and adhere to this schedule so that you can rest daily.

- The same mood regulation in biochemistry also controls nutrient appetite, which influences the function of neurotransmitters such as dopamine and serotonin, which are essential in anxiety and depression. This means this your appetite can be deregulated according to your mood, so you will most likely be annoyed when you fast.

- The last suggestion for individuals involved in an intermittent fasting diet just restricts the alcoholic intake during eating hours. Do not drink alcohol during or just after fasting, and even if you eat, bear in mind that drinking alcohol will reduce your chances of proper nutrition.

CONCLUSION

The diet you're trying to adopt when Intermittent Fasting is going to be decided by the outcomes you're searching for and where you're starting, so take a look at yourself and ask the question what do I expect from this?

If you're looking to lose a substantial amount of weight, you 're probably going to have to take a closer look at your diet. Still, if you just want to lose a few pounds on the beach, you could find that a few weeks of intermittent fasting will do it for you.

For women who are interested in weight loss, intermittent fasting can seem like a great idea. Still, many people want to ask, should women be fast? Is intermittent fasting successful for women, right? There have been a few primary studies on intermittent fasting that can help shed some light on this fascinating new dietary phenomenon.

Intermittent fasting for women has several beneficial effects. What makes it particularly important for women who are trying to lose weight is that women have a much higher fat content in their bodies. When trying to lose weight, the body primarily burns through the first 6 hours of carbohydrate storage and then begins to burn fat. Women who have a balanced diet and exercise schedule may be dealing with stubborn fat, but fasting is a practical solution.

Intermittent fasting may not be a good idea for every woman. Anyone with a specific health condition or who tends to be hypoglycemic should consult a physician. However, this new dietary trend has unique benefits for women who naturally store more fat in their bodies and may have difficulty getting rid of these fat stores.